"This book provides answers to the most important question mental health professionals ask when learning how to work with children: How do I actually do it? With great clarity on the purpose and methods associated with a wide range of play therapy activities, this book truly integrates play into the therapeutic process. It treats play as a form of expression, a natural home for assessment, and an avenue for effective intervention. The creative exercises detailed in this book will be useful in any child therapist's toolkit."

Benjamin E. Caldwell, *PsyD, LMFT,*
Adjunct Professor at California State University, Northridge, USA

"A Must-Read for Family Therapists! An essential resource for family therapists, *Creative Play in Family Therapy* offers practical strategies for seamlessly integrating creative play into traditional family therapy. The interventions are not only effective but also deeply engaging for children, making therapy sessions more productive and enjoyable. A game-changer in the field!"

Diane Gehart, *Ph.D., Founder and CEO,*
Therapy that Works Institute; Professor Emerita at California State
University, Northridge, USA

Creative Play in Family Therapy

This practical resource integrates family therapy theory with playful interventions and techniques to allow family therapists to successfully engage and include children in the session.

Many therapists who are trained in family therapy lack training in child-centered play techniques. This book effectively bridges the gap between popular theories and models in family therapy and the practice of working with children in a family context. Showcasing playful therapy techniques across and within each of the most common models of a family therapy, such as Experiential, Structural, and Narrative Therapy, and Psychodynamic and Cognitive Behavioral Therapy (CBT), this book is accessible to a wide range of clinicians. Additionally, the author offers clear tangible interventions adaptable for both in-person and teletherapy sessions.

This book is essential reading for practicing therapists, students in training, clinical supervisors, and anyone who works with children in a therapeutic capacity.

Lisa René Reynolds, Ph.D., is Assistant Professor at The Family Institute at Northwestern University, as well as a licensed therapist in Connecticut and New York.

Creative Play in Family Therapy

Effective Strategies and Interventions for Child-Centered Treatment

Lisa René Reynolds, Ph.D.

Routledge
Taylor & Francis Group
NEW YORK AND LONDON

Designed cover image: Getty Images

First published 2025
by Routledge
605 Third Avenue, New York, NY 10158

and by Routledge
4 Park Square, Milton Park, Abingdon, Oxon, OX14 4RN

Routledge is an imprint of the Taylor & Francis Group, an informa business

© 2025 Lisa René Reynolds

ISBN: 978-1-032-82765-0 (hbk)
ISBN: 978-1-032-82763-6 (pbk)
ISBN: 978-1-003-50607-2 (ebk)

DOI: 10.4324/9781003506072

Typeset in Times New Roman
by codeMantra

Contents

Acknowledgments

A book like this could not have been created without acknowledging the incredible group of kid clients and their families that I was able to practice and hone my playful therapy skills on. You were all a great audience and I learned so much about the art of playful therapy from and with you.

Thank you to my professional peers and colleagues for support and companionship on this always-evolving road of being a competent therapist. My gratitude goes out to the student "therapists-in-training" who have been so grateful to learn tools and incorporate playfulness over my many years of teaching and supervising—thank you for your eternal interest and hunger!

Thanks to my editor, Julia Giordano, for her support and interest in this topic, and for her belief in my ability to create an important guide. Thanks also to the Routledge team who also believed in this important work and made the writing journey painless.

My biggest gratitude goes out to my incredible family, who have always supported everything I do. Thanks especially to my parents who encouraged my writing early on, my three amazing adult daughters who are my everything, and to my "partner in the final chapter"—I love you all!

Introduction

Tell me and I forget. Teach me and I remember. Involve me and I learn.

~Benjamin Franklin

This famous quote is linked often to the importance of using play in therapy with children. "Tell me" is what traditional therapists did many years ago; their directive and interpretive training led to a more instructional type of therapy. "Teach me" certainly has a place in the therapy room, but with children it is not always an effective strategy without creative and playful efforts. However, "involve me" is especially poignant in working with children in a way that helps create and grow foundational changes that will serve the children we see for the rest of their lives. *Play* is the conduit for involving children in the therapeutic process.

There are many registered play therapists (RPTs) who practice around the United States. In the two states I am licensed in there are 16 (Connecticut) and 42 (New York), as per the Association for Play Therapy (APT). However, there are scores more (psychiatrists, psychologists, social workers, family therapists, practical counselors, and school professionals) providers who offer therapy to children, teens, and their families every day who do ***not*** have play certification. Furthermore, when one searches for registered play therapists who also speak Spanish in New York, for example, that number drops from 42 to 4. In short, there are a limited number of certified RPTs, and even less of them who speak languages other than English. So where does the play training come from for the average, non-RPT therapists who see the bulk of youngsters in practice? And is the play training adequate to meet the needs of child clients?

Many therapists (counselors, social workers, marriage and family therapists) I know do not feel that they had adequate training in playful interventions in graduate school. Most report learning strategies through experience and "trial and error" or from CEU workshops they chose to attend. Additionally, it has been my experience as a graduate school professor in therapy training programs that the younger generations of therapists lack the ease of being creative with playful ideas for working with youth. These newer generations of therapists grew up

DOI: 10.4324/9781003506072-1

with many more "screens" opportunities, resulting in less experienced practice in creative "free play."

Creative ideas for play may come easier to their older counterparts who grew up spending their days playing make-believe with dolls or action figures and exploring the neighborhood in search of something fun to do.

Play is universal, and is relevant for every child in any sort of therapy around the world. Meta-analytic reviews of research aimed at examining the efficacy of play therapy on positive outcomes in work with children (e.g., Bratton et al. (2005); Jensen et al., 2017) are plentiful. Play therapy is linked to successful outcomes over and over again, especially when parents are involved in the treatment, making it a great fit for systemic therapists who work with children in the context of other relationships (e.g., family, siblings, and peers). However, relatively few therapists go on to complete the intensive training of the registered play therapy path, and therefore practice without the specialized training.

I have observed countless videos and live sessions of therapy trainees working with younger clients, and the most frequent pattern I see is of "play—therapy—play—therapy." In short, therapists will often play with kids in treatment, then stop the play and attempt to ask standard "therapy" questions, and then return to play. This is problematic in a couple of ways. First, when the kids get a "taste" of playing in a session, they can be reluctant and maybe even irritated or resistant to being asked to do "therapy." Of course playing is more enjoyable than thinking and answering therapeutic questions! Second, the "play—therapy—play—therapy" method can feel disjointed and hard to stay on a therapeutic track for both therapist and child when fun distractions enter the work.

Since the pandemic resulted in many therapists moving permanently to remote teletherapy services, creative and playful therapeutic techniques have become even more difficult to provide. I have provided classes, trainings, and playful therapy labs for graduate students for many years, and each one is met with such overwhelming gratitude, excitement, and participation from trainees. Attendees report the easy, straightforward, and simple techniques and interventions to be of infinite usefulness in their therapy sessions with children and families.

This book aims to help therapists to do therapy *playfully* with younger clients as the baseline of the entire session, rather than the more typical taking turns of playing and doing therapy during the session. Additionally, many interventions will offer suggestions for adaptation to remote/teletherapy, which can be particularly challenging with younger children. Each chapter offers a model-based overview with tangible, practical, playful interventions that therapists can implement in their therapy with children and families. Admittedly, each chapter takes a creative pathway, geared toward younger minds and concepts and activities, toward each model's basic tenets. However, the outcome of playful-based interventions that adhere to foundational models of therapy is rewarding. Perhaps the most valuable part of creating a space full of playful therapeutic interventions for young clients is that they can take these lessons and tools with them throughout life. Although the actual game or emotional drawing activity might not be used in the adult years, the message that those activities hardwire into young clients will remain there forever. These powerful internal messages can be drawn upon throughout time.

1   Structural Therapy

Model Background and Key Concepts

Structural Therapy (e.g., Minuchin, 1974) is one of the original models in the field, with Salvador Minuchin as the founder. He created the model while working as a psychiatrist at the Wiltwyck School, a home for inner-city delinquent boys. During his work there, he discovered that traditional psychoanalysis proved insufficient treatment for change. He began to experiment with systemic therapy, treating the boys *and* their families, and prioritizing the live observation of their interactions.

This model focuses on clients' issues existing within faulty structure and alignment in their family and/or other relationship systems. When working with children or families, a therapist using structural techniques would focus on things like boundaries, hierarchy in the system, where things like triangulation, alliances, or coalitions exist between people, and roles and other system expectations. Structural Therapy works well with families, but can also be used effectively with individuals or with social, peer, school, or work issues.

The therapist using these structural techniques would view the client(s) through the lens of—*clients are part of a structural "system," meaning that they are viewed as recursively influencing each other.* They do not create issues in a vacuum. From this jumping-off place, the following are some of the techniques therapists can use.

Playful Technique Ideas

Joining

This is an important focus of *all* models. Joining involves the therapist making connections and relationships with clients to meet them where they are and form a trusting alliance. It is aimed at increasing comfort levels that will create a safe space and assist in the opening up process during sessions. The main way to join while beginning the work of Structural Therapy is to bring the idea of everyone

DOI: 10.4324/9781003506072-2

being part of a *system* to the forefront. We *care* about the others in the picture and how they contribute to, reinforce, or maintain the presenting issues.

During the initial intake, be sure to ask questions that include a focus on the "system" surrounding the client you are meeting with. For example, if you are meeting with a child and a parent, be sure to ask for the views of *both* parent and child on things. If you are seeing the child alone, you can check in periodically with questions like, "Do you think mom would agree with that answer?" or, "Does your sister feel the same way?" or, "Can you think of any of your other friends who might be surprised by how you feel about that?" This is a very subtle way of ensuring focus on the *systemic* nature of how we view the existence of any one client's presenting problems.

"Mimesis" is one way that Structural therapists join with the family. That is, therapists will maintain their roles as active participants or "members" of the system (family) by matching the style of the family to fit in and be part of it. Examples might be using the language or tone or speed the family uses in conversing, joking around with the family if that is part of their interactions, etc. When working playfully with a child alone, the therapist can remain part of the client's system by dramatically acting out the parts of other family members or the child's friends or teachers. Therapists pretending to be the client's mom might attach a sticky note to their shirt with "MOM" written on it and change their voice to match the mother's tone. Then, the therapist and child can rehearse discussions the child might have with the parent and prepare for the different ways the conversation might go.

Mapping

Mapping involves a therapist uncovering information and data points to help figure out where the interactional patterns exist. From this information, the therapist can make decisions on how to proceed in therapy.

• Drawing out a family tree or "genogram" is a playful way to map a child's system (see also the Bowen Therapy chapter for more ways to use the genogram). The difference between a family tree and a genogram is that the genogram takes it a step further and includes the relationships between people and interactional patterns and highlights things like enmeshment or cutoff. Additionally, genograms can show things like divorce and death, which opens up areas of conversation that can be helpful in understanding the context of the child's life.

Therapists can also use this tool to highlight a child or teen's social group, including labeling peers as "leaders" or "followers." Including lines to represent closeness, distance, conflict, or cutoff between members can be a great visual for the clients. Variations of the genogram can include using action figures, animals, or cut out waiting room magazine images to represent peers or family members. These figures or images can be lined up or spread out on the table or the floor, and members can be moved around as needed. For teletherapy, the therapist can share the screen and look for different online photos or the child can share their camera roll of family photos.

Remember that Structural therapists care about things like hierarchy, roles, and proximity, so some great questions to ask a child while creating the setup might be, "Wow, so it seems like this one friend of yours is always connected to the drama with the others, huh?" or, "I noticed that your mom has conflict lines with everyone else in the family." These activities can be adapted for teletherapy very easily, especially for younger clients who will enjoy drawing pictures or arranging figurines and showing and explaining them to the therapist through the online platform.

- Boundaries are important to explore in the mapping stage of Structural work. Also, boundaries are such an important tool to teach children, teens, and families about, *especially* when there are issues with abuse, neglect, trauma, and other interpersonal distresses. Teaching about and practicing boundaries with children lends itself well to playful interventions.

Colored masking tape (royal blue painters tape works really well and is an inexpensive staple for the therapy room) can be used to make a hands-on and visual representation of the concept of *boundaries*. The therapist can tear off pieces of the tape and have the child stick the line of tape down on the floor between family members to show where the limits of overstepping are. If the child is seen alone and the therapist has done a family or social network genogram, colored markers are great for drawing boundary lines between people represented there.

Another playful way to talk about boundaries is for the therapist to move closer and closer to the child or teen in the room and have the client express how close the therapist can get before "it gets weird." Questions like, "So what were you feeling inside when I got this close to you?" or, "What are some things you could do or say to me if I got too close?" are great to use.

- Hierarchy is also an important theme to map in clients' relationships. One of my favorite playful strategies is to use a toy car as a prop and ask the young client, "Who's driving?" This can be used to acknowledge that a parent makes the rules, or that a child doesn't have to follow what another kid is doing at school. Another way to highlight the concept of hierarchy when working with a family is for the therapist to have the kids make a "crown" out of construction paper and pass it to whichever family member is speaking to wear. Glue or a glue stick and a shoe box with an assortment of fake jewels, stickers, and embellishments are great things to have on hand in the office for this activity, as well as many others contained in the book. For teletherapy sessions, the therapist and child or child and family can co-create a Power-Point slide with various words to describe family organization and roles on it, like "leader" or "peacemaker."

Unbalancing

This involves a therapist briefly aligning with a certain family member to address gridlocked behaviors and perceptions to promote changes in behaviors. In person, therapists can physically move around the room to get closer to one specific family member. Other ways to unbalance or "shake up" the family "stuckness" are to ask members to role-play each other in an argument or discussion. A child may role-play the mom and say, "You are a very bad child and you make me really mad and I don't love you anymore!" This can be playful and light in some incidents but can also give a new level of understanding of how family members view each other. In this case, the child's view of mom not loving anymore is a powerful thing and a great opening for the therapist to prompt mom to dispel the misunderstanding.

Another strategy to use with a solo child or a child and family, is to play the "What if..." game. The therapist can introduce the idea of things being "stuck" in a certain, undesirable way (e.g., fighting, disagreeing, "attitude" or anger) and ask a series of questions for the client(s) to imagine. An example would be if the client reported his mother being rigid and punishing and unfair and the therapist responded, "What *IF* you told your mom that's how you felt? Let's imagine how would you feel *telling* mom you feel that way. What would her reaction be?" Another example would be the therapist saying, "What *IF* you tried something different? What would happen? What big, bold move could you make on your part that would get a happier response from your mom?"

Another great way to "play" with unbalancing is using classic board games like Don't Tip the Waiter™ or Don't Spill the Beans™. These games are very hands-on, and don't take very much attention, so they are generally not very disruptive to the therapeutic process. Both games challenge players to pile items onto the waiter's hands, or pile beans into a pot without them tipping over. The therapist can label the pot as the child, and try to figure out what "beans" (e.g., "a mean kid at school" or "a teacher who is mean") add up to the child feeling "full" or overwhelmed. "Beans" (e.g., "playing with friends" or "looking forward to weekend plans") can be removed to help the pot feel lighter and more stable when there are more positive things to focus on. Likewise, the waiter game can have each hand represent a person in a dyad (e.g., the child and the parent) and put items on each side to represent stressors or good things. The therapist can then discuss questions like, "Who 'wins' and who 'loses' in certain situations?" or "Who do you think has the most dishes piled on when you have an argument?"

Reframing

This involves altering the way an event or situation is perceived by offering a different perspective and challenging the family to consider it as an opportunity to look at things differently. The "art" of reframing lends itself beautifully to playful intervention. This activity is especially good for children who struggle with being hurt easily, are overly sensitive, or personalize others' actions, and those who act bossy and judgmental.

First, therapists can talk about different things that people like to set up in the context of "reframes." For example, the different kinds of ice cream flavors people like or how some people like to live where it's hot and sunny and near a beach, while some prefer a cold Alaskan fishing village or a bustling European city. Next, the therapist can ask the child where would be the best place to live and why. Then the therapist can open up the reframing, or pretending to answer from other people's perspectives. To make it more fun, the therapist can use different voices to represent different people or can invite the child to chime in for rationale others might have for why they live where they live. So for example, the following are some examples of people's responses to wanting to live in a particular place:

- "I'd **_HATE_** to live where it was hot all the time! I hate being sweaty and would miss having a fireplace and not being able to go sledding or skiing!"
- "I'd **_HATE_** living where it's cold all the time! I'd miss swimming in the ocean, feeling the warm sun on my back, being able to ride my bike all the time, and having cookouts in the backyard!"
- "I'd **_HATE_** living in a big city! It's so noisy and dangerous and there's always traffic. In a big city you can't see all the beautiful stars at night and you don't have a fenced backyard for your dogs to run around in!"
- "I'd **_HATE_** living in the country! You have to drive so far to get to places when you live there and you might not have any neighbors nearby. I'd be bored and lonely in the country!"

Next, the therapist can introduce other ways that people might think. For example, if the child complains that this girl (Jazmin) at school is really mean and bossy, the therapist might "reframe" the statement with one of the following options:

- "I wonder if Jazmin thinks she's being mean or bossy, or maybe that's just the normal way members of her family act with one another at home?"
- "Do you think maybe Jazmin's 'bossiness' is really something else? Like, maybe Jazmin thinks there are better ways to do things and just tries really hard to get others to see it the same way she does?"
- "I wonder if Jazmin being 'mean' might really be that she's just feeling really angry about something and so it comes across as 'mean?' What are some things that might be going on in Jazmin's life that could make her feel angry? Being left out? Having friends that aren't nice to her? Feeling bad about herself?"

Teaching children the art of "possibilities" in cognitive reframing can be an incredibly useful, lifetime tool. After doing some of this work with kids, I will frequently ask the child in subsequent sessions with different scenarios about what another possible view on something might be. For instance, "So how do you think your mom would explain how your argument went with your sister last night?"

Reframing is especially well suited for teletherapy as well. A simple internet search under "images" for the term "picture frame" will yield countless choices. The therapist can keep a few screenshots of these images to include in making a slide that can frame any number of photos, words, or situational write-ups that the client provides. Another way to do this is to search famous artwork and look through some art online together and talk about which ones the therapist and client like or dislike and why, as well as the *why* someone else might like/dislike it. Also, it's helpful to add a discussion of context—a loud, vibrant, dark, ominous-looking piece of artwork might not fit in a newborn baby's bright yellow nursery, but the same art might look great in a haunted house or an edgy, modern hotel.

Enactment

This involves a therapist helping to facilitate a role-play scenario and act out certain situations to come to a better resolution. Enactment takes the form of *action* over talking. Simply talking *about* situations often lacks the experiential piece of actually being *in* it. The following are some playful ways to introduce the usefulness of enactment with child clients:

- Perhaps the easiest way to introduce enactment is to regularly instruct the child or family members to directly talk to each other in session instead of to or through the therapist. If the child is seen alone, the therapist might say, as the child is complaining about how his brother hogs the gaming system, "If your brother were here right now, sitting next to me, talk to him, tell him how you feel about the fairness of the gaming time." The key is for the child to *tell* what he feels and would say safely in the therapy room, rather than the less action-oriented talk *about* the situation. This serves as both a chance at rehearsing the situation that will inevitably take place again sometime in the future, as well as give the therapist, in live-time, the opportunity to intervene, suggest, or "coach" the live interaction. This exercise also gives kids the chance to act out and rehearse the interaction which may make it easier to happen more organically when a similar situation pops up at a later time.
- Seat arrangement is a classic Structural Therapy staple. The therapist can ask family members to move seats in session to demonstrate alliances, subsystems (like sibling groups), or closeness of family members. The therapist can direct a client to go sit next to his brother so the two can argue about what they think the fair rule should be about who gets to use the video gaming

system at what times. The Structural therapist might coach the parent(s) to interject or explain to the children if they agree with what they are proposing. Many children learn and understand best when they can look at a visual of something.

Parentified Child

In some families, it becomes evident that there is a child who has been given or taken on the role of "parentified child." A parentified child role means that the parent gets emotional support or physical help from a child, rather than giving it. In this role reversal, we might see a young boy worried about his stressed-out mom (because she regularly vents to him about how much she hates her job) and so he barks at his siblings to stop fighting and tells them to be quiet so mom can sleep. Additionally, he might take on the extra task of cleaning up dishes after dinner or helping a younger sibling with homework so that the mom doesn't have to.

- The therapist can help the child client draw, color, and cut out some objects that represent a "grown up" or "parent" and others that represent a kid. While talking about family interactions, the therapist might interject and challenge the child by asking, "Hey, so is that a kid thing or a parent thing you're doing when you clean up your sister's room?" Another variation the therapist can use to raise the client's insight and awareness is to just grab the grown-up "item" (maybe a picture of a colorful tie to wear to work) and put it up to themselves silently to indicate the label of "parent" or "child."
- Another helpful and playful way to address the parentified child role is to write up a "prescription" (you can buy fake, blank, colorful ones online, or ones with preloaded check boxes like, "Take a walk," or, "Be kind to yourself" on them) that states, "You are given permission to be a child right now." The therapist can include the parent(s) or guardian(s) in this powerful activity by having them sign it under the therapist's signature.

There are many ways to use the tenets of Structural Therapy in playful ways with child clients and/or their families. Using these interventions can assist clients in understanding the concepts in meaningful and developmentally-appropriate ways. Additionally, the techniques described above can realign family structure and interactions, and supply clients with tools they can take with them into future situations.

Case Example

The parents bring their three children for therapy with complaints that the fighting at home has "gotten out of control." The family consists of two dads, their twin seven-year-old daughters (Kylie and Kelcie), and their older (adopted) brother, 11-year-old Rafael. The family is upper middle class and white, except for Rafael who was adopted after a foster placement fell through when he crossed over the Mexican border alone four years previously. The dads report that Kylie and Rafael are close and that they pick on Kelcie ruthlessly. They also share that the kids think the dads favor Kelcie and are easier on her with rules in the household.

A Structural Therapist's Intervention by "Clarisse"

The therapist, Clarisse, joins the family by asking each member why they are there and what they want to get out of therapy. After hearing their responses and learning a bit more about how they each view the problem, Clarisse then asks the girls to come sit on the floor next to her and asks Rafael to sit in a chair across the room, and directs the dads to move together on the small couch.

Clarisse then asks a series of questions to the family, including things like, "Who is the most in charge of the family?" and, "Who is the softest in the family?" She then asks the two girls to turn to one another and talk about a recent argument they had about whose turn it was to use the Wii. As they are arguing, Rafael interjects with, "Kelcie is such a liar! She's so greedy with everything, she's spoiled, and NEVER lets anybody else use stuff!" Then the dads chime in, defending Kelcie with, "Stop being mean, Rafael! Your sister is NOT spoiled or a liar, that's just mean to say that!" Clarisse stops the girls and turns to Rafael and the dads and says, "I'm going to have you all do a task for me while I'm listening to the girls enact their fight." She hands out pads of colored sticky notes and pens to everyone and asks them to write down the labels that come to mind for other family members. *Liar. Spoiled. Mean.*

Then she takes her roll of blue painter's tape and tears off pieces to make a box around the girls on the floor. "We are going to try something different. This is the talking box. I'm going to have all of you take turns coming into the box with other family members and only when you're in the box can you talk, okay?" Then Clarisse tears off a piece of tape and puts it on the floor in front of the dads, and another piece on the floor in front of Rafael. "Everybody is going to try to maintain a boundary here and stay behind their line. Physically and verbally."

As soon as Clarisse directs the girls to return to their discussion, Rafael speaks out again, "You're so bossy, Kelcie!" Clarisse walks over to Rafael and says, "I feel like that is a big burden for you to have to always be mediating and being the parent in this situation. I'm going to ask you to just be an 11-year-old right now." She hands him a pair of multicolored squishy balls and continues, "How would it be if I asked your dads to take over right now? So you don't even need to pay attention or listen for the next ten minutes?" "I think you're too young to take on dad duty at 11, don't you?" Clarisse jokes with Rafael, since she gauges that the family does use a bit of sarcasm and humor in their interactions. She then moves over to the dads and says, "I want you both to just *listen* to the girls. No need to say anything. You can take notes if you want to say something afterward, okay?"

While listening to the girls, Clarisse quickly assesses that the issue between them is really rooted in competition and bad feelings. Kelcie appears "favored" by the dads and this makes Kylie angry and jealous. Kylie is "favored" by Rafael and this makes Kelcie hurt and feeling left out. After the girls finish, Clarisse has Rafael and Kelcie enter the "talking box," followed by the dads and Kylie.

At the end of the session, Clarisse shares her thoughts on the family dynamics with everyone. She asks them to each take a homework assignment for the week. She sends the dads home with one of the squishy balls and instructs them to give it to Rafael and tell him he has permission to leave the room and "go be an 11-year-old" when fights break out. She also asks the dads to make a concerted effort to spend time with both girls together. The girls are given a playful activity to do together during the week to get to know each other better (create ingredient lists for the best and worst pizza toppings and then decide on which ones they will make with the dads for their regular Friday family dinner). The sibling dyad of Kelcie and Rafael are also asked to do something together, and they decide on Rafael teaching her a new video game.

Lastly, the therapist collects the sticky note labels that the family created and holds onto them for the next week. She also sticks a piece of the blue tape to each person's hand to take home and use as a "boundary marker" if someone is saying something that angers or upsets them. If any family member produces the blue tape, the others are to think about what they are feeling and rather than argue, they can go write it down in the family notebook that Clarisse has suggested they keep in a central area. She asks them to bring the notebook into the next session so they can discuss.

Key Takeaways

Structural Therapy will always center on a few key concepts when using the model in playful interventions. The following are a few key elements to remember when working from a Structurally-informed lens:

- The *structure* (How is the family made up? What do roles and boundaries look like? Where can we see things like triangles, alliances, or coalitions people between people?) and *function* (patterns of interaction) of the family are essential basics to always keep in mind when using this model.
- Explore everything "systems." When a client issue is presented, we want to focus on who says/thinks what, and then what they do, and then how others respond, and generally how it all lays out.
- When looking to explore how functioning occurs, inviting enactment between clients gives the therapist the best, live, in-action view into those interactions.
- When clients/families seem "stuck" in cyclical patterns, the role of the Structurally-informed therapist is to unbalance or "shake up" the stuckness.

2   Strategic Therapy

Model Background and Key Concepts

The foundational contributors to Strategic Therapy (e.g., Madanes, 1981; Haley, 1976) include John Weakland, Don Jackson, Paul Watzlawick, and Richard Fisch. They based their thoughts on the earlier work of Gregory Bateson and Milton Erickson. This chapter will infuse a bit of Mental Research Institute (MRI) and the Italian Milan Group models as well, since all three were created along the same vein of early systemic treatment. Although all three have their own distinctions and hallmarks (you'll discover some of those in the following text), they all use similar processes.

This model focuses on how clients' issues exist within family and/or other relationship systems. When working with children or families, a therapist using strategic techniques would focus on things like homeostasis, family rules, breaking patterns, and figuring out in what ways the client(s) has tried to fix the issues that haven't worked and become problems of their own.

The therapist using these Strategic techniques would view the client(s) through the lens of—*people resist change, symptoms have a function and purpose, people often contribute to problems via their own failed attempts at solutions.*

The following are some of the techniques therapists can use with young clients that utilize the basic tenets of Strategic Therapy.

Playful Technique Ideas

Family Rules

Every family or system has their own set of "rules," some that are spoken, and others that are not. It can be helpful to assist children in uncovering some of these rules to help them better navigate situations with others. A fun activity with families can be for the therapist to stand at a whiteboard and write down the family rules as members share them. It can add helpful context for parents to share some of the rules that were the same or different when they were kids growing up.

DOI: 10.4324/9781003506072-3

Different colored dry erase markers can be used to represent different family members' rules. For a teletherapy variation, the therapist can share a screen to create the document using different colored fonts, and a copy can be emailed home and printed out for the family to reference or make notes on.

Another layer of this task might be to talk about what happens when someone "breaks" a rule, or whose responsibility it is to enforce the "rules." This can uncover things like a parentified child, common feedback loops that occur in the family, or help to define and clarify unspoken "rules."

Consider this segment of a session with the therapist, the 14-year-old client Emi, and her mother:

Therapist: Emi, what are some of the big family rules you can think of that you have in your house?

Emi: Well, *that's* easy! We cannot, under *any* circumstances, talk about our feelings in this family.

Therapist: I'm going to write this "rule" down on this piece of paper (*The therapist writes, "Cannot talk about feelings."*).

Therapist: Mom—any thoughts on this?

Mom: Well that's ridiculous, of *course* we can talk about feelings!

Emi: That is *so* not true, Mom! If I dare talk about how I feel, *especially* if it's different from the way you want me to feel, it's shut right down.

Mom: You don't understand, Emi…you can feel differently than I do, and I accept that you have feelings that are different from mine, but it's the *way* that you say things that I shut down. I don't like being sworn at or yelled at or accused.

Therapist: So, let me see, maybe we have to change this family "rule?" (*The therapist crosses out the first statement and replaces it with, "We can express feelings, but there are certain ways that we are expected to do so."*)

Breaking down and clarifying family rules can help clients better understand expectations and this helps the therapist formulate goals for treatment. In the scenario above, the therapist sent both Emi and Mom home with a sticky note of the better-defined "rule" of expressing emotions.

Attempts at Resolution

Strategic therapists center their work on the belief that clients' own actions, and *especially* those intended to "fix" the situation, may not only *fail* but also become problems themselves and exacerbate the initial problem sequence. The following clinical example of a single dad (John) and his 17-year-old daughter (Imani) complaining of a constant pattern of fighting about household rules demonstrates how one attempt to fix a problem (John telling Imani what he needs her to do differently) has turned into a secondary problem:

Therapist: John, hold on…can you turn to Imani and tell her a bit more calmly what it is exactly that you need her to do differently? Take a minute first if you need to…

John: (*sighs loudly*) I guess…but I ALWAYS talk to her about it, curfews, talking back, swearing, using a vape, and it goes in one ear and out the other. It never goes anywhere, and NOTHING ever changes.

Therapist: So it seems like we have *two* problems here—one is the fighting about household rules, and the other is this pattern that when you talk, John, you feel like Imani doesn't listen to you and that your communication never changes anything, is that right?

One of the most helpful ways that therapists can assist child clients and their families is to understand that (failed) solution attempts can sometimes create *additional* problems. Deciphering between the two can help clients to create different sets of skills to deal with each "problem" rather than just growing one problem bigger by adding the fallout from failed attempts at solutions for it. The following is another way that therapists can help child clients understand problems and responses to the problem that can create *more* problems.

A therapist's favorite is to draw a "decision tree" that begins with a question like, "How does an argument happen in your family?" and then offers subsequent questions like, "Who starts the argument?" and, "Then who responds to that?" and, "And who decides when the argument is over?" The Milan-influenced therapist would call these questions "circular questions" that are aimed at highlighting the circular nature of patterns of communication rather than a more linear view of simple cause and effect.

The therapist can then move into putting red Xs or green √s next to each question to note whether the action helped or didn't help the situation. You can order stickers of the Xs and √s or rubber stamps and stamp pads to have a more hands-on approach for younger children. For online sessions, you can use the "advanced symbol" option or "picture" and then "stock images" and "icons" on your Word toolbar to get different variations of Xs and √s.

A further use of the actions that get an "X" for not being helpful to solve the problem or the green "√" is to write them down separately on pieces of paper and clip them together with a fun clip (online you can purchase inexpensively, all different shapes and colors of paper clips or tiny binder clips). Perhaps using a red clip for the red X "not helpful" pile and a green clip for the green "√" helpful pile will be helpful for younger children to remember. The therapist (and maybe the parents if they are involved in the session) can help the child generate more "√" options for things to do differently that might yield a better outcome in changing the argument.

"Go Slow" Messages

It may seem counterproductive, but since Strategic therapists generally believe that the problem has some function in the family, simply trying to get rid of the symptoms is not the first goal. This is where the "go slow" message can come in handy. The therapist can "prescribe" that the client and/or the family not give up the problematic issue yet (e.g., arguing) because they may not be ready to deal with the turmoil that losing that important piece might bring on. The arguing serves a purpose and carries some important message. This is also an example of what Strategic therapists would call, "perturbing the system." In short, "perturbing the system" means doing anything that raises the intensity and "shakes up" what the client or family is doing. Oftentimes, making the problem worse can cause a shift in the interactions, thus changing the problem's presentation. Blank "prescription pads" can be ordered online, or therapists can simply use different colored and shaped sticky notes to write the "prescription" for client/family to take home as described in the vignette below.

Consider the following clinical case with the therapist using perturbation and the "go slow" messaging with two moms, and their nine-year-old child:

Therapist: Okay, so you all have pretty much agreed that there is a lot of fight-ing in your household at bedtime, right? (*Both moms and the child nod in agreement*). And I know you all came here to try to *stop* the arguing and make bedtime go better, but I'm thinking that we need to be *very* careful about just removing the arguing altogether. That would be a *big* change, and I'm not sure we are all ready to prepare for what comes with that. So bear with me on this, okay? (*The thera-pist grabs a blank prescription notepad and writes the following: The family will plan to have one argument every night about the bed-time routine, but you will have it directly following dinner instead of at bedtime, and you will all wear your pajamas and have the argu-ment sitting in a circle on the bathroom floor.*) Now, does everyone agree with this?

The therapist has effectively warned the family not to expect the problem to go away immediately, but rather to embrace it and give it someplace in their interac-tions, but to do it in a different way. Should the client or family return the follow-ing session having had an argument, then they had been warned to expect and invite it. However, if they return with a report of no arguing or less difficult bed-times, then this will be a welcomed event all around. Either way, it's a win-win!

"One Cannot NOT *Communicate"*

Strategic therapists really highlight that "one cannot **_not_** communicate." What this means is that even silence, a stoic facial expression, crossed arms, a sigh or a snort, or leaving the room carries *some* meaning. These actions or expressions communicate *something*, and it's important to help clients and families understand this. Non-verbal communication is so powerful, especially to younger clients who make the most sense of the world and meaning by things like body language, facial expressions, actions, and sounds. Clients or family members may not accurately guess what those things are meant to communicate, but rather, come up with their own ideas of meaning. This can cause problems in the child's interactions with others.

This concept is especially important to use very young children who might not have much experience with others' actions and what they mean, or with neurodivergent children or those with attention deficit issues that may not be able to recognize or focus well on others.

Some playful ways to demonstrate this with child clients is through role-playing different people in the child's life (family members, friends, teachers) and using different body language, facial expressions, and sounds to explore the meaning and possible "messages." For family sessions, members can playfully describe or act out how they know when another family member is mad or sad or hurt. For an online variation, the therapist can share screen and search for images of different facial expressions or body language (e.g., crossed arms, tight posture, turning away) and discuss what possible "messages" those people in the picture might be sending (e.g., I'm angry, I'm uncomfortable, I don't want to be here, I'm scared, I'm hurt by you).

Consider the following clinical vignette with the therapist, a dad, and a 14-year-old son, Rafael:

Therapist: So Rafael, you keep talking about how dad is so disappointed with you all the time. I'm wondering if you can share with me *how* you know he's disappointed?

Rafael: Oh, I know when he's mad and disappointed. Because it's like, *all* the time!

Therapist: Okay, but I want to know *how* you know that.

Rafael: Because he has this mad face and scrunches his hands up in fists and looks at me with disgust.

Therapist: Can you show me what that face looks like, Rafael?

Rafael: (*Rafael stands up and acts out his father's typical reaction*)

Dad: (*Laughs*) Rafael, that is *not* what I do! Yes, I might look mad because I *am* mad, but I don't get why you think that means I'm disappointed...

Therapist: Dad, did you know that's the face you make when you're mad? And did you know that your son interprets it as mad and disappointed?

Dad: No, I didn't...

Therapist: Rafael, so how do you feel about the next time your dad makes that face and has that stance, asking him if he's mad or disappointed or both? And dad, maybe you could tell Rafael when you're feeling angry that that is all it is, and that disappointment in him is not what you are expressing?

When I have used this intervention with families, there is often a "lightening" in the room when members act out themselves or each other. Sometimes there is even laughter, or a commitment to try to be more aware of certain facial expressions. You can keep a large hand mirror in your therapy room and family members can try looking at themselves when they are feeling certain ways in session.

"One Down" Position

The "one-down" position can be a powerful tool to use in session. This position is a tactic that helps the therapist control the room by taking a stance of helplessness, confusion, or unknowing. This allows the client and/or family to become the "experts" and offer insight and explanations.

Examples of one-down stances for therapists to take in order to "perturb" or shake up the system might include:

- Hmmmmm...I'm a little confused here. I thought we all agreed last session that keeping the arguments in place was probably a good idea, but now you're saying there weren't any arguments this week?
- I guess I was a little quick to jump the gun so to speak...I think it was maybe premature to ask you all to do the arguing differently this week.
- Maybe I was wrong in my assumption that you all really wanted to minimize the arguing...maybe it has a much more important role than I gave it credit for in your family.

Using the one-down stances allows the client and/or family members to take the lead and address and explore issues that the therapist has creatively laid out for them. This can lead to a shift in the family's interactions, discussions, behaviors, or understanding of each other and the "problem."

First-Order vs. Second Order Change

First-order/second-order change is a concept that is incredibly helpful for children to understand. First-order change is an action or thought that temporarily shifts the dynamics in a system (or family), but with practice, those shifts can become more permanent and actually become part of the system's habit or regular functioning. Some examples are as follows:

- Mom starts using gold stars to reward son for cleaning his room (first-order change because Mom has employed a new strategy to change the dynamic of arguing over household chores, but not yet second order because we don't know if the son's efforts improved and that this became the new, more successful "dance" in the family).

- Parents try several strategies to get their daughter to come home on time for her curfew (first-order change, ditto from the above explanation).
- Parents negotiate rules with son on things like extending curfew or letting him take on responsibilities now that he is 17 years old (Second order change because the parents have understood and accepted the changing role of parents to an older teenager and as such, have instituted an organic mindset that allows for different rules in the family).

When working with children and/or families, using numbers (you can make your own cut-outs from construction paper, or order number stickers or dies online) is a great way to label separate problems. A fun "game" to use with child clients is to ask them to choose the cut-out of "1" or "2" to label things that happen in family or peer group interactions as either, (1) A new, temporary effort, or, (2) A deeper, regular change that has solved something more permanently. Consider the following clinical case with two brothers who are always fighting:

Therapist: So you two say you are *always* fighting? But now you've decided to just stop talking to or playing with each other altogether to fix the problem, huh? (Both brothers nod in agreement).

Therapist: So this "solution" of not talking to or playing with each other seems to have temporarily solved the "problem" of fighting because you are no longer in the same room or space to have a fight, right? (Again, both boys nod).

Therapist: (*Taking out a shiny, red cutout of the number "1"*) So this staying away from each other is a temporary fix. (Therapist writes, "stay away from each other" on the whiteboard and affixes the shiny number "1" next to it). But what about the bigger problem of why you two can never get along? If we put you in a room together, the fighting would start again, no? (*Both boys nod*). Hmmmmm….(*The therapist writes the original problem on the board, "always fighting," with big question marks after it*). So, what do you think the solution to the actual problem of fighting is? (*Boys shrug and simultaneously state, "I don't know."*).

Therapist: Well, I have some ideas, so maybe I can throw a few out and you two can let me know if you think they might be part of what's going on.

Content vs. Process

All clients can benefit from understanding the difference between "content" and "process." "Content" is the "stuff" clients come in talking about. "Process" is what's underneath that "stuff." Therapists are trained to be mindful of not getting caught up in the (often very interesting or entertaining) "story" the client is telling, but rather to focus on the "process" of what's going on underneath.

For example, 12-year-old Perry tells you, "I don't want to go see my dad on the weekends he's supposed to have me. He's mean and I don't like him. He yells all the time and he's always mad at me." The "content" is about a mean dad who is always mad and yells all the time. The "process" is the "stuff" underneath. The following questions are some examples of what the therapist might ask Perry in order to delve into the "process" behind dad being mean and yelling and mad. Since different models of therapy might inform the various questions the therapist might ask to uncover "process," I've included the model in parentheses after each example:

- "So Perry, what's going on right before dad gets mad? (Perry answers, "I usually ask him to do something that he says 'no' to.") "Are there ever times when you ask dad to do something and he surprises you by saying, 'Yes?' [Narrative (see more in Chapter 8) "Unique Outcomes" or "Exceptions" in Solution Focused Therapy (see more in Chapter 7)]"
- "So when dad says, 'No,' Perry, then what happens next? (Perry says, "I get mad.") And then what does dad do when you get mad? And then what happens next?" ["Circular Questioning" from Milan/Strategic]
- "Perry, tell me about how you feel inside when dad yells at you..." [Experiential Therapy]

If children are old enough to understand the difference between the story told ("content") and what's going on behind it ("process"), it's great to explore frankly about it with them. However, if children cannot easily understand these concepts, I keep several laminated "story cards" on hand to share as examples with my younger clients. For example, on an index card, I print out a short story on one side (content):

Marika hit her brother and called him a jerk and said she hated him because he stole the rest of her Halloween candy from the bowl in her room and left the empty wrappers strewn on her floor. On the other side of the card (process), I print: Marika is angry because her brother took one of her special things without asking. She is frustrated because she has asked him not to take her things before and she doesn't know how to make him stop doing it. She's told on him to her mom but the stealing stuff without asking still doesn't stop. So Marika hits him because she's so angry at him and hopes that maybe that will scare him into stop taking her things without asking.

The therapist can create similar "story cards" with child clients in session (this works for teletherapy as well) with the "content" on one side, and the "process" on the other side to refer to at home next time the situation happens. Clients can also share these with parents or siblings to help collectively understand the problem (Marika's frustration with her brother for taking her stuff without asking) and possible failed solutions (Marika telling her mom on her brother or hitting him).

Odd Day/Even Day

This intervention can be a big hit with child clients and families alike. It's a very simple assignment! When there is disagreement in the family or arguments over the way to do things, etc., the therapist can ask the client or family members to try doing different things on different days of the week. This is a good step toward clients *trying* something different, when they are not ready or willing to fully take on a different way of doing things. Consider the following clinical case from my practice with ten-year-old Shaniqua and her mom:

Mom: She (*Shaniqua*) is not allowed to play outside with her friends until *after* she finishes her homework. She has a problem with always saying she'll do it, and putting it off, and putting it off, and then never doing it.

Shaniqua: Mom! That's not true! I know that's what I've sometimes done before but it's getting darker earlier and I *promise* I'll do it, but I just want to play with my friends before I have to come in...

Mom: Shaniqua, you've promised me this before and you didn't do it.

Shaniqua: But I like to do my reading and journaling at night before bed anyway. I *always* read before bed, you know that! So why can't I do the math stuff before I play and then the reading and reading journal before bed? That's fair!

Mom: I'm not playing these empty promise games with you anymore, Shaniqua! What do you think, Dr. Lisa?

Therapist (a.k.a. "Dr. Lisa"): Well, I think you're the mom and you are trying to do what's best for Shaniqua's schoolwork and her learning. I also think that Shaniqua seems really motivated to strike a both/and deal with you where she does some homework, plays outside with her friends, and then finishes up reading and journaling before bed. But I also know that her track record hasn't always gone so smoothly. So I'm wondering how you feel about trying an experiment this upcoming week. So on "even" days, Monday, Wednesday, and Friday, Shaniqua will do her Math and other assignments as soon as she gets home from school and then goes out to play, and then is ready for bed at 7:30 and does her reading and journaling and is ready for lights-out by 8:15? And then on "odd" days, Tuesday and Thursday, Shaniqua will do all of her homework as soon as she gets home and before she is allowed to play outside. What if we try that out and see what happens? Next time we meet, we can talk about how things went and then decide on whether Shaniqua's plan works, or if we need to go back to doing it another way.

Letter Writing

Letter writing is intended to transfer the work that occurred in the therapy room beyond the meeting by reminding the client(s) to continue things that occurred in the therapy session after they leave. This is an especially great technique to use with younger child clients, who enjoy getting their very own mail or messages. Even with older child clients, teens, or families, a reminder email message or a fun mailed message can be both exciting and a useful reminder of things the client (hopefully) is thinking about or trying or doing differently outside of therapy.

The following are two examples of messages I sent to clients between sessions. The first was a short, handwritten message on colorful cardstock with cute designs on it, printed in glittery marker that was snail-mailed to a nine-year-old. The second was a group (encrypted) email sent to a 16-year-old client and his parents.

#1:   Jamie's Job for the week: When you want to yell mean things at your mom, ask yourself first, am I, (1) Mad, (2) Embarrassed, or (3) Hurt. Then just yell, "I'm mad!" or, "I'm embarrassed!" or, "I'm hurt!" instead of the mean things you would normally say.

#2:   Hi Burress Family! Just a reminder that in the last session, you all decided to try some things a little differently. Checking in with:
   Dad: Had said he would try to not jump into heated discussions with son and instead, lean into mom and work together on how to address together.
   Mom: Had said she would be truthful with dad about how she felt about his ideas and when they decided on a plan, she would support him on it.
   Son: Had said he would try to be patient with hearing his parents out and then take time alone to reflect before he responds to them.
   I'll see you next week and look forward to hearing about how the week went!

Rituals

Rituals are one of the easiest and most helpful strategies to use with younger clients and/or their families. They can be very effective in helping clients move on from people, events, or actions or feelings from their past that they are ready to let go of.

One of the simplest ways to use rituals is to have clients write down something from their past that they have "conquered" in therapy and are ready to dispose of. I keep a box of scraps of colorful paper and a myriad of shapes and colors of sticky notes in my office. Have the client write something like, "Hitting my brother" (when the behavior has ceased) on a scrap of paper, and then scribble over it in black marker, or crumple up or rip up into pieces, and throw it into the trash can in the office.

One of my favorite examples was an activity I did with a five-year-old (Maya) many years ago. This was a child who had very low self-esteem and often concerned her grandmother (the guardian) by saying things like, "I'm stupid," or, "Nobody likes me," or, "I'm bad," or, "I hate myself." After many months of work with this client, she was much more positive about herself. On our last session together, I picked a daisy from the grass near the parking lot in my office and gave it to her. I plucked off the first few petals and said things like, "Maya is loving and kind to animals," and, "Maya is a really big helper in the kitchen," and, "Maya is a very good friend." After each statement, I threw the petal up into the air where it floated off and fell to the ground. I asked her to finish off the rest of the petals with positive statements about herself and told her that she could ask her grandmother for help if she needed to remember more.

Years later, I bumped into Maya in a grocery store. She spotted me and came up to me and told me that she was back home from college for summer break after her junior year. She told me that she never forgot the flower and that she still practiced the ritual of reminding herself of her positives when she was feeling down. She said that since she rarely had a flower handy, she did it with peas on her dinner plate, pens on her desk in her dorm, or when washing dishes. The "ritual" that was so fun for a five-year-old with a daisy, became a much larger lesson and strategy for the client that she carried with her into her adult life.

Again, for teletherapy clients, many of the techniques shared in this text can be done easily. The therapist can send a few supplies (like scraps of paper or sticky notes) via snail mail to the client, or direct the client to find such things around their house to use. I have occasionally asked a parent or guardian (if they have the time and money to do so) to make a fun outing with the child to pick out some "therapy supplies" like a fun notebook, stickers, or colorful sticky notes. This is especially helpful in making therapy an enjoyable and engaging activity for young clients who might otherwise become bored or disengaged, especially via remote sessions. It is super easy to ask a teletherapy client to go out in the yard and pick a flower to use for the ritual.

Case Example

Eleven-year-old Kai and his twin brother Keanu are brought in to see the therapist, Eliana, by their parents. The parents share that the fighting between the brothers has just become "out of control" and that they need help navigating what to do about it. Eliana decides to employ a Strategic approach to the family's issue.

A Strategic Therapist's Intervention by "Eliana"

After hearing each person's description of the problem, Eliana points out the failed solutions that have created new problems for the family. Then, she uses circular questioning to highlight the recursive patterns of the family's interactions. Lastly, she decides to give the "go slow" message to the family and follows this with several directives, aimed at "perturbing" the very "set in stone" patterns the family describes.

Therapist: Okay, well thank you all for the detailed descriptions of how this all goes down in your family. I feel like I have a pretty good understanding of how things seem to go at home. It seems like there might be more than one problem going on here though. So, we have the fights that Kai and Keanu get into that start as yelling but then get physical. And you all report they are happening more often lately. But then when the fights start, mom usually gets involved and then things seem to get worse, right? Then dad gets involved and then things get even worse. Hmmmm...so seems that not the boys, or mom, or dad are able to do anything to stop the fighting, but rather, all the attempts to make it stop make it actually *worse*. I'm going to ask you all to help me out here with something. Can we talk about the fight over the last piece of pizza last night? I'm going to start and then hand the "talking stick" to one of you and I want you to tell me, step by step, what happened next, okay? (*Family nods.*)

Therapist: Okay, so the dogs start barking and dad walks in the front door with two pizza boxes in his hands. (*Hands the talking stick to dad*).

Dad: Kai runs over and grabs the boxes to try to help me take them to the kitchen.

Therapist: Can you hand the talking stick to someone else now, dad? (*Hands to Mom*).

Mom: One of the pizza boxes fell off the top and out of Kai's hands and fell upside down on the floor and a few pieces fell onto the carpet. (*Hands to Kai*).

After a few minutes when everyone has contributed to the multilayered details of the prior night's events, Eliana sums up what she heard from them, and describes the several problematic issues that seem to have come out of the interactions (placing blame, making assumptions, using profanity, saying hurtful things, physicality). Next, she says,

> You know, I think there's a lot here and I don't think we should try to make it all change overnight. So let's slow things down and just see how this next week goes, but let's anticipate that there will be another fight, and I think we should be ready to figure out what purpose it serves in your family. This next week, I'd like for you all to be looking for when the fight is starting and I want you all to make space for it. Sit around the table together and just like we did with the talking stick today, take turns "stating your case" with one another by handing off an oven mitt instead of the talking stick. Are you all on board with this?

Some therapists are uncomfortable with using the escalation and perturbance techniques of this model, but I'm including them here because I have seen others use them with positive results. I too have used such techniques on occasion with certain families and found them to be beneficial.

Key Takeaways

Strategic Therapy will always center on a few key concepts when using the model in playful interventions. The following are a few key elements to remember when working from a Strategically-informed lens:

- Clients often contribute to their problems via their own failed attempts at solutions. These failed attempts are an important thing to look for throughout therapy, as they may serve as roadblocks to therapeutic progress and change.
- One cannot *not* communicate is an important tenet to remember. For this reason, one goal of Strategically-influenced therapists is to explore and challenge particular words, attitudes, postures, or body language that serves to communicate *something* that may need to be probed further.
- Problems serve some purpose. For this reason, it's vital that Strategically-informed therapists respect and leave space for how the problem may hold an important role in the client's life.
- The one-down position is a helpful one for therapists according to this model. This means that being "confused" or curious or otherwise asking for clients' help in understanding their issues can be beneficial stance for eliciting the best outcomes in treatment.

3 Bowen Family Therapy

Model Background and Key Concepts

Murray Bowen is the central figure in the creation of Bowen Family Therapy (e.g., Bowen, 1966). Michael Kerr and Edwin Friedman are others often cited in the early work with this model. This model centers on the notion that clients often perpetuate their issues by attempting to fix them in ways that fail and then become problems themselves.

This model focuses on several assumptions such as symptoms existing as signs of stress or anxiety, the concept of differentiation, and the powerful transmission of "rules" and "messages" from one's family of origin. Additionally, Bowen Family Therapy stresses the importance of educating clients about these concepts, detriangulating, and using genograms and process (or thinking through) questions as ways to assist with change and decrease in symptoms.

The therapist using these Bowen techniques would view the client(s) through the lens of—*change occurs and symptoms improve when anxiety is reduced, and clients are able to become more differentiated.* They do not create issues in a vacuum. From this jumping-off place, the following are some of the techniques therapists can use.

Playful Technique Ideas

Differentiation

Differentiation is a key concept in the Bowen Model. It focuses on the two "poles" (togetherness and individuality) that are always at play for each of us. Too much of either can have negative and stressful consequences. It can be a difficult thing for children to understand, so the following are some playful ways to help children work on differentiation.

- The therapist can explain that we each have two "places" in ourselves—one is togetherness and one is being alone. If children are being seen in person, the therapist can put a piece of paper with "together" on it on one side of the floor

DOI: 10.4324/9781003506072-4

and another with the word "alone" on it on the other side of the floor. Clients can move back and forth between the two pieces of paper, sharing times when they are around others (maybe at school or a family dinner), and times when they are by themselves (in bed at night, being the last one left sitting in the back of the school bus). The therapist can help clients express what they like and how they feel when they describe the times alone or with others.

Too much "togetherness" can cause unhealthy fusion or lack of being able to be oneself, so the therapist can ask questions to assess whether this is an issue:

- When you are hanging out with that group of kids on the playground, do you always do what they do, or do you get to choose sometimes?
- When your family is fighting, do you ever have anything to say? If I were to be listening in on your family fighting in the kitchen one night, would I hear your voice in there?
- When it's time for you to leave the family interactions and go to bed at night, are you sad or upset to be by yourself?

Likewise, too much individuality can cause a lack of emotional connection, feeling left out, or even cutoff. The following are some good assessment questions for therapists to ask their child clients:

- When the kids are playing on the playground, do you ever wish you could go join them?
- What would it be like to go sit downstairs with your brothers while they're playing video games?
- Can you imagine asking someone in your class to be your partner when the teacher assigns an activity?

Genograms

The previous chapter utilized the genogram tool a bit to lay out the structure of a family system, however, the genogram is most often linked to the Bowen model. Unlike a simple family tree, the genogram goes deeper, exploring things like relationships and boundaries between people, where fusion, cutoff, and enmeshment may occur. For use with child clients and/or their families, the genogram is such an incredible therapeutic tool to use.

- Therapists can create genograms on a whiteboard, posterboard, or on simple copier paper. For remote adaptation, therapists can use the whiteboard screen option on their platform or there are several online sites that offer free customizable genogram templates that the therapist and client can do in session. Conversely, as a family homework assignment, the therapist can send the family home with a blank, hardcopy template to complete together, using a different color marker or pen for each family member's contribution. Another kid-friendly touch you can use is having the child add labels for people in the family by asking questions like, "Who is the nicest in the family? Who is the angriest? Who is the quietest? Who is the peacemaker?"

Family Emotional Processes

Bowenian therapy is interested in how emotional processes and beliefs are passed down and kept alive throughout generations. The genogram (see above) is a good place to start to explore where messages may have been transmitted down from grandparent to parent to child.

- While looking at the genogram with a family, the therapist can facilitate discussions about what the generational messages are for each family member and how those may shape how family members feel about themselves and others. For example, consider the following dialogue between the therapist, a young client, and the client's mom:

Therapist (to client):	Hmmmmm…so you think that mom yells all the time and expects you to be "perfect?" Tell me a little bit more about why you think that.
Client:	She yells at me for everything. Like if my bed isn't made *perfectly* or I'm like *one* minute late getting up in the morning.
Therapist:	So I wonder if you know anything about how Mom's mom parented her? Do you know what your grandma expected of your mom when she was your age?
Client: No.	I don't remember my grandma. She died when I was like three years old or something.
Therapist (to Mom):	So Mom, can you tell us a little bit about what life was like at home with doing stuff around the house when you were your child's age?
Mom:	Sure! I get that it was different times back then, but my mother worked two jobs to keep a roof over our heads and food on the table. She expected us to help out and we did what she asked, *when* she asked, because we were grateful for what she did for us. We wanted to help out to make life easier for her.
Therapist (to client):	Aha! I think I figured something out about your mom! We all kind of learn how to parent from what we get from our parents when we were kids. So it seems like your grandma worked hard and expected her kids to help out as a recognition and "thank you" for what she did for them. Do you think that mom expecting you to show appreciation by doing chores and being on time and listening to her was something that was passed down to her from her mom?

Client:	I guess that's probably true.
Therapist (to mom):	So maybe it isn't really about the bed being made perfectly, but rather that you are looking for things that show appreciation for all the things you do to help your child?
Mom:	Exactly. I just want to feel appreciated.

The therapist could then engage the client and mom in a discussion about expectations and chores and appreciation. Additionally, the assignment of homework would help carry the new interactions home with them:

Therapist (to client):	So I have an idea for homework for you this week. Every time Mom wants you to ask to do something, I want you to try to remember that doing things her mom asked her was how she showed that she appreciated her mom. Then I want you to think about what you appreciate about your mom and what things you could do to show her that.
Therapist (to Mom):	And Mom, I want you to remember that there are lots of ways to show appreciation and maybe you can spend this week looking for the different ways your child is grateful. Maybe the "thank you" might not come in a perfectly made bed, but maybe they will be shown in different ways than how you were expected to show your mom you appreciated her.

Another favorite intervention to use with kids on this topic is what I call the "Who Am I?" game. Therapists can have the child clients draw a picture of themselves on a piece of paper and decorate it as they wish. Next, the therapist has them write different family "messages" they received on sticky notes and attach them around the paper drawing of themselves. Examples might be things like, "You should always respect your elders," or, "Good people are kind to others." When they are done, the therapist asks them to share what those messages mean to them and decide if they want to "accept" or "reject" each one. In other words, do they want to carry those messages on with them and pass them down to their own kids? Perhaps a child client will explain that "Good people are kind to others" is both accepted *and* rejected. Further exploration yields that the child feels that yes, being kind to others is a good thing, but there are certain times when someone might *not* be kind to someone else, and that doesn't make that person *bad.* This activity can be done easily in a family session as well, with all members present creating their own "Who Am I?" drawing with their family messages attached accordingly.

Triangles

Triangles are not *good* or *bad* according to this model, but rather, they are just something that people do to manage anxiety. One of the goals of Bowen's work is to decrease the anxiety in a system and detriangulate where possible. When working with child clients, it's important to point out and explain triangles.

- Again, the genogram is a great way to point out and draw in triangles. The therapist can use stuffed or small plastic animal miniatures to form relationships between people and then demonstrate how triangles happen. For example, let's say the therapist is seeing a ten-year-old boy who is having social issues at school. The boy complains that every time he plays with this other kid at recess, as soon as the other kid gets bored or wants to play something different, the kid goes to the teacher and tattles that the client is being bossy and won't let him play the game he wants to. The therapist would then ask the client to choose two animals that represent both him and the other kid. The therapist would have the boy act out the playground scene with the chosen animal figurines and then would introduce a third animal (ideally one that is bigger and more adult-looking) and form a triangle between the three. Some good exploring questions for the therapist might be:

  - "How do you think you and the other kid could handle this in a way that the teacher didn't have to be triangulated into things?"
  - "What do you think this other kid needs in order to not need to go get the teacher's help?"
  - "How do you think going to the teacher helps this kid feel better?"

Process Questions

Process questions are used in this model to simply help clients *think* about things so that they might be better prepared for navigating them. I like to keep a small stack of notecards (laminating them makes it easier to wipe them off and reuse endlessly) that have process questions written on them. The therapist can presort appropriate questions and have the child client choose a couple of the cards to respond to after sharing a difficult event with the therapist. Examples of good process questions might be:

- "What do you think about that?"
- "How do you think doing that will work out?"
- "How was that for you?"
- "What was your interpretation of mom and dad's discussion?"
- "What do you think the short and long-term results will be of you not doing that anymore?"

Sibling Position

Although some more post-modern therapists shy away from Bowen's work on sibling position, I still find it helpful to explore the powerful experiences of siblings in some child sessions when the dynamic seems pertinent. It can be helpful for children to understand that a sibling's birth position might have an influence on how they experience things in the family or might contribute to the traits they embody.

- The therapist working with one child might ask questions about how the client's siblings might experience certain events differently. For example, the therapist might ask, "So do you think your older brother felt as scared as you did when your dad got angry and yelled?" or, "Why do you think your dad yelling didn't seem to bother your brother as much as it bothered you?"

Managing Anxiety

The Bowen model centers on the concept of anxiety and how it contributes to problems. Interpersonal conflict, dysfunction within a person, or triangulation are common ways that people deal with anxiety. Reducing emotional reactivity is an integral part of helping clients increase thoughtful, calm responses in interactions with others.

- Therapists can help young clients understand the management of anxiety in a myriad of ways. First, the therapist can draw two circles on a whiteboard (or on the remote platform whiteboard for teletherapy clients) and label them "thoughts" and "emotions." Teaching the child how these two are different is a foundational piece of managing anxiety. For example, ten-year-old Alex comes in for therapy with you, complaining of having issues with friends and his brothers. As Alex tells his story, the therapist can write things like, "embarrassed" or "anger" in the feelings circle, and "I don't like how I never get a chance to say how I feel" or "He *always* tries to control things" in the thoughts circle. Separating the two can help the client to see how feelings are simply that—*feelings*—and thoughts are things that can be explored and reframed, leading to reduced anxiety.
- Bowen also highlighted that when we can plan out how we want to respond, it makes it easier for us to practice how we will respond in situations, thus lowering the level of anxiety we experience. Role-playing is a great way to help children practice the ways that they might show up differently in situations. Consider the flowing dialogue between the therapist and ten-year-old Alex (above) who shares issues with his friends and brothers:

Therapist (using process questions):	So when you are arguing with your brothers and you tell me that they "always win," what do you think about why that is?
Alex:	They just always "win" because they don't listen to anything I say and never let me have my way with *anything.*
Therapist:	Hmmmm…so you have *thoughts* about how they interact with you, but how does it *feel* when they don't listen to you?

Alex:	It makes me really, really mad and feel left out.
Therapist:	How do you feel about practicing what you could say to your brothers when situations like this occur? How about I will be your brother and you can practice telling me how you feel?

Case Example

Kaia is a 12-year-old African American female who lives with her single mother, Patricia. She is described as an "overachiever" at school, and recently Kaia's teacher reached out to Patricia to suggest she take Kaia to see a therapist. The teacher reports that Kaia has recently begun picking at her nails until they bleed and frustratedly jabs her pencil into her leg if she gets an answer wrong in class. She has been acting angry and glaring at the teacher in class as well. She has also started to pick on another girl in class by mocking her for being "dumb" and not doing her homework and getting answers wrong when the teacher calls on her. Patricia agrees to take her to see someone and reports that she has noticed that Kaia cries more easily lately and has been having a hard time falling asleep at night and has been complaining of "tummy aches" that the pediatrician thinks are anxiety-based since the tests he ran came back normal.

A Bowen Therapist's Intervention by "Manny"

Manny meets with Kaia solo for the first session, and crafts a genogram with her, complete with labels for all the people on it. Kaia labels her mom as "demanding" and her "absent" father as a "deadbeat." Interestingly, Kaia labels herself as a "perfectionist." Manny jumps on Kaia's description of mom as "demanding" and explores what "demanding" looks like in her family. Manny quickly separates what "demanding" looks like versus how Kaia feels when she thinks that her mom has demanding expectations of her ("sad" or "not good enough").

Manny talks about the ways that Kaia embodies anxiety. He explores Kaia's awareness of picking at her fingers and stabbing her leg. He then coaches her on ways to calm anxiety, and has her draw a picture of herself with the parts of her that feel upset when she's dealing with her brothers or peers circled. Again, Manny focuses Kaia's descriptions on how she *feels* when these events are occurring and rehearses with her how she could navigate her frustrations verbally or physically in the classroom.

Manny then tries to help Kaia detriangulate the teacher and the other girl in the class from how Kaia feels. Manny asks her, "Who cares if that girl does her work or get the answers wrong? How does that girl's answers to questions impact you?"

Manny asks Kaia's mom in the next session to explore the messages she received growing up on being a "good student" and the expectations she has for Kaia on what academic success looks like. Manny is careful to place the focus on the *message* of what "success" looks like, rather than on either Patricia or Kaia. Consider the following dialogue:

Therapist: So Mom, it seems like academic "success" is something you want for Kaia?

Mom: Of course!

Therapist: Was this an expectation your parents had of you as a child?

Mom: Absolutely.

Therapist (to Kaia):   What do you think about doing well academically?

Kaia: It's so important if you want to go anywhere! You can't be stupid and not study and answer questions wrong.

Therapist: So you don't feel good about getting answers wrong? Tell me how getting a wrong answer makes you *feel,* Kaia…

Therapist: So when you think your mom is demanding better of you, what could you say to her to let you know you understand?

Kaia: I'm doing the best I can, Mom!

Therapist (to Mom):   Can you help Kaia understand both your expectations, like keeping up, doing her homework, and getting good grades and the feelings you have towards your daughter, regardless of her academic performance?

Mom: Sweetheart, you are a good student. I want you to be successful in school so you have an easier life than I had. It's not about what the teacher expects or what other students do or don't do. I just want you to try your best and not be upset if you don't get things perfect.

The goal of the therapist here is to decrease the emotional reactivity of the client (Kaia) and to have her understand the expectations that were passed down in her family. Manny also wants to help Kaia understand how she is *feeling* and how that influences the way she acts towards others in situations at school or at home. Additionally, he wants to expand the options of how Kaia can show up in situations with others. He attempts to detriangulate the teacher and other girl from the expectations Kaia feels are put upon her, and to redirect those feelings towards a better understanding of her family's emotional processes and how she embodies and acts on her anxiety from these.

Bowenian therapy offers a number of areas to focus on when working with child clients and/or their families. The model lends itself to playful exploration of family dynamics and labels, utilizing genograms, categorization games for separating thoughts and feelings, and strategies for decreasing anxiety and emotional reactivity.

Key Takeaways

Bowen Therapy will always center on a few key concepts when using the model in playful interventions. The following are a few key elements to remember when working from a Bowenian-informed lens:

- This model focuses on the assumption that clients' symptoms exist as signs of stress or anxiety. Finding ways to heighten awareness of, and decrease levels of these is paramount to good Bowenian treatment.
- Bowenian-influenced therapists recognize the powerful transmission of "rules" and "messages" from one's family of origin and keep these as a central focus of therapeutic exploration to uncover their role in problem identification and problem-solving.
- Bowen therapists stress the importance of educating clients about all of the model's concepts (e.g., triangulation, differentiation)
- Bowenian-influenced therapists find great importance in creating genograms with clients/families, and using process (or thinking through) questions in their work with clients.

4   Contextual Therapy

Model Background and Key Concepts

Ivan Boszormenyi Nagy is the founder of Contextual Therapy (e.g., Boszormenyi-Nagy, 1987). The model centers on the notion that trust and health in relationships emanates from repeated occurrences of ethical and fair interactions. If relationships are *not* trustworthy, entitlement and "debts" start to build up and need to be "paid back." People keep emotional "ledgers" of unfair actions, and these "unbalanced" ledgers must somehow get "balanced," many times in ways that are destructive to clients and their relationships and often to future generations.

This model focuses on how values are passed down through generations, how split and individual loyalties drive people's motivations and behaviors, and the impact of these on not only the here and now, but also on future interactions across subsequent generations.

Playful Technique Ideas

The Four Dimensions

The four dimensions is a tool that young clients can carry with them forever. The four dimensions are facts, psychological, relational, and ethical. Whenever a client is looking at a problem, it is helpful to sift through these four areas before deciding how to tackle it. When I had an on-ground practice, I kept four laminated index cards, each one with one of the aforementioned words on it. So imagine that eight-year-old Katie comes to your practice for issues with being bullied at school. The therapist could explain the activity, and then lay the four cards out on the floor (or hold them up to the screen for teletherapy), asking about each one. This also gives the therapist the opportunity to add ideas to the categories that might help the client see things a bit differently. Here are some examples that Katie and the therapist might come up with:

- Facts: *Some* kids say mean things to Katie and make fun of her curly brown hair and freckles; Katie does have very curly brown hair and freckles.

DOI: 10.4324/9781003506072-5

- Psychological: Katie feels embarrassed when the kids tease her about her appearance, Katie feels angry at those classmates who tease her, Katie feels "ugly."
- Relational: Katie can identify two kids in her class who don't bully her, Katie is shy and doesn't really talk much to other kids, and teachers are generally really nice and kind to her.
- Ethical: It doesn't seem fair that when the teachers hear the other kids say things, they don't tell them to stop, it's not fair that the kids pick on her hair and freckles when another girl in the class has *way* curlier hair and *way* more freckles.

The facts of a situation, how we feel about it, the interactions between people, and the perception of fairness are not all the same things. Helping a child to understand the difference between these categories and making a practice in therapy of calling out things that might be in the wrong category can be a useful practice. One example might be when Katie lists a "psychological" feeling of "being ugly," the therapist might help her understand that "ugly" is how Katie *feels* when the kids note her hair and freckles, but it is *not* a "fact." Furthermore, the therapist might help Katie to expand the list of "facts" to include, "I'm not ugly," as evidenced by things Katie likes about her appearance and what she hears from other people and what she thinks when she looks at pictures of herself. "Ugly" is just a *feeling*, not a *fact*.

Loyalties

Two types of common "loyalties" that make for solid clinical work with young ones are "split" and "invisible." Split loyalties can be found in the typical divorcing parent scenario for children or in social competition between friends. In the case of parental divorce, this is where a child might feel torn between the parents, and carries the stress of feeling bad or siding with or being angry at one or both of them.

Consider this segment of a session with the therapist, the nine-year-old twin clients (Arla and Starr), and their mother (who is in the process of divorcing her wife, Diane, the children's stepmother):

Therapist: So girls, Mom tells me that you two used to have a great relationship and were like "best friends" to each other. She says that recently, you two have pulled away from each other to "take sides" with either Mom or Diane.

Arla: Starr is stupid! She acts nice to Diane and hugs her when she comes over but Diane is a bad person and Starr should be mean to her.

Therapist: Arla, can you tell me why you think Diane is a bad person?

Arla: Diane is mean to Mom and makes her cry all the time. Diane moved out and left Mom with all the work.

Therapist: Mom—any thoughts on this?

Mom: Well, it's true that I have been crying a lot lately. But that's because I'm sad and stressed out, Arla. But Diane moved out because one of us had to and it made more sense for me to stay in the house since I'm home with you girls more.

Therapist: Starr, tell me what you think about all the changes in your family.

Starr: It's not Diane's fault Mom cries all the time. Arla should feel bad for Diane because she lives all alone now and misses us and Arla should be nice to her. Arla is the one who is a bad person because she's so mean to Diane!

Therapist: So, let me see, it seems like you girls have different thoughts on this and feel like you need to protect or take care of or stand up for either Diane or Mom…

Therapist: Mom, let me know if you agree with this, okay? Arla and Starr, can you both come sit on the floor with me and help me make some paper cut-out dolls of your family members? (*The therapist helps the girls draw and color in paper cutouts that resemble themselves, Diane, and their Mom.*)

Therapist: So let's talk about what happens when Diane comes over to visit. (*Therapist picks up the Diane cutout.*) Who goes to greet Diane? (*Starr picks up her own cutout. The therapist then adds a colorful, sparkly paper clip to hold the two cutouts together.*) And where is Mom when Diane comes over?

Starr: She goes into the other room and Arla follows her. (*The therapist picks up the Mom and Arla cutouts and clips them together.*)

The subsequent conversation centers on the therapist asking about each child's loyalty to protecting a parent and what it would take for Starr and Arla to be able to give themselves permission to just be sisters and "best friends" again and letting Mom and Diane work things out between them. The therapist invited Diane to join the session the following week and gave the homework assignment to each of them to be "clipped" to another person; Arla to Starr, and Mom to Diane. With help from the therapist, each dyad gave an "assignment" to the other; Mom and Diane were supposed to clean the kitchen together, and Arla and Starr had to help each other clean their hamster cages.

"Invisible Loyalties" are when there is a "secret" or hidden reason why a client favors one person over another. The unspoken nature of these loyalties can cause problematic undercurrents and patterns of interactions between family members. For example, if Arla believes that Diane favors Starr and that Starr is her favorite child, this may be part of the motivator for Arla to be angry toward Diane. One of my favorite therapeutic activities (this can be done in the office, or at home for teletherapy clients) is for the family to create a posterboard for each family member. The clients can either draw a picture of each family member in the center of each poster or print out a photo to tape in the middle. The family members can each write positive things about each other on the posters. Things like, "kind" or "loves animals" or "has a beautiful smile" are a few ideas. This activity can begin to dispel gently any myths about favoritism or alliances.

**Note: For parents who have a difficult time coming up with "positives" for a child who is showing a lot of anger and problematic behaviors, the therapist may help guide the parents on how to phrase traits as positives. Some examples might be "energetic" for a child who is overly active, or, "Curious" for a child who is always getting into everything, or, "precise" instead of "perfectionist" for a child that has some obsessive-compulsive tendencies. There are many sites online that can give you more ideas on alternates for trait descriptors.

Entitlements/Destructive Entitlements

We can all make decisions on what we deserve by judging the worthiness of others and how we perceive them to treat us. These are "entitlements." They're not inherently "good" or "bad," but rather, just *are*. For example, 12-year-old Juan Carlo tells the therapist,

> My dad doesn't like me very much. I'm *always* doing something wrong in his eyes. That's why I don't like to see him except when I *have* to, like on holidays. My stepdad is more like a real dad to me. He's nice and talks calmly about stuff if I do something he doesn't think is okay.

"Destructive entitlements" however, can be more damaging to both clients, as well as their relationships. Destructive entitlements show up when people feel like they were "slighted" or have had bad things happen to them, so they feel that because that wasn't fair, it's okay to pass along negative energy to others because of it. So for example, let's take 12-year-old Juan Carlo again. The following would be an example of destructive entitlement:

> My real dad has been a jerk to me my whole life. I don't like seeing him, and he shouldn't even get to be a dad because he just sucks at all of it. He yells at me and I can never do anything right. So when my stepdad tries to tell me to do something, like clean my room or turn off my video games, I tell him to eff off, because he's not my *real* dad and doesn't get to tell me what to do.

A playful way to utilize these concepts further with minor clients is for the therapist to ask two questions regularly to help the child if it is an entitlement or a destructive entitlement. The first is, *"Does this help you?"* And the second is, *"Does this hurt you?"* Helping Juan Carlo to see that getting angry with his stepdad for typical parenting requests that are done calmly and respectfully might *hurt* him because it might stand in the way of him having a healthy, loving relationship with his stepdad as a "father figure." Destructive entitlements show up here as rigid responses to the stepdad that end up destroying the healthiness of that relationship because there is a history of Juan Carlo being treated poorly by his biological father.

Ledgers

"Ledgers" are the proverbial way we "keep score" of what others do to/for us. It's the balance of these things that make us feel good, like the relationship is "fair." "Balancing" these ledgers is a key goal in Contextual Therapy.

Good games to have on hand in a therapy office used to see minor clients are Don't Spill the Beans™ or Don't Tip the Waiter™. In these games, objects (beans or dishes) are piled up until they fall. This is a good way to help children understand ledgers and how things "pile up." Another idea is to use a double-pan balance scale where the child can put pieces of paper with things written on them on the scale, with each side representing a separate person in the relationship. Is the scale "balanced?" What needs to happen to make the two sides feel more "balanced?" These are good beginning questions to ask child clients and/or their families in session to highlight how ledgers work.

Actions

Contextual therapists adhere strongly to the notion that healthy "bridges" *between* people are built by *actions*, more than by thoughts or feelings. For this reason, therapists might want to encourage young clients to explore what they can *do* about things they discuss in therapy sessions.

If we take Juan Carlo again, with his frustration with his biological father's poor treatment of him, the therapist could approach the discussion by opening up spaces for Juan Carlo to figure out how he could handle things differently with his dad and stepdad. Questions like, "Have you ever talked to your dad about this?" or "What do you think dad's response would be if you told him how you feel?" are good openers. The therapist can have Juan Carlo write on an office whiteboard (or on sticky notes at home for teletherapy clients) a list of specific examples of what his dad has said or done that made him feel this way. After each item, the therapist can help Juan Carlo figure out if there is anything he could do to make the outcome turn out differently. For example, Juan Carlo writes, "My dad tells me I'm lazy," and then after it, writes, "It makes me feel bad when you call me lazy," or, "Yes, I put off doing my homework sometimes, but it's because I procrastinate, not because I'm lazy."

"Homework pads" are a great staple for therapists who work with young clients and/or their families. You can order pre-printed ones online, or you can print your own with checkboxes and spaces to write in "action items" for clients to *do* between sessions.

Right Script-Wrong Player

Sometimes, we have the right idea of what we need, but we might go to the wrong person to try to get that need met. This is in essence the idea behind Contextual's "Right Script-Wrong Player." In clients' attempts to "balance" the unfair "ledger," they may sometimes look to the wrong person to fix things. Consider the following vignette between the therapist and a (divorced) mother-daughter (Cleo) duo:

Mom: Yes, I'm angry, Cleo! You're right, I *did* yell at you last night because I'm sick of you making messes and just assuming I'm going to take care of them.

Therapist: Tell me about what happened last night, Cleo…

Cleo: I got home late. Dad dropped me off like at 9:30 pm and I had to get up for school in the morning so I didn't have time to do my laundry. So I just dumped out my suitcase in the laundry room and left the empty suitcase in the hallway to go back up in the attic. I was gonna do those things today but instead she [Mom] came screaming at me in bed this morning and I was so exhausted.

Mom: Yeah, I'm *sure* you were exhausted, Cleo. Poor *you.* Dad took you away for a week on a fancy Caribbean vacation and I'm sure you're *so* tired. No one told me when you were getting home, or that it would be that late, and it must be nice for dad to do vacation but not have to deal with the piles of laundry and snippy, exhausted daughter afterward.

In this vignette, there are two things going on. First, there are some expectations from Mom of daughter that need to be parsed out—where to dump laundry? Rules on timing of doing laundry? Keeping in touch regarding the estimated time of arrival after being away for a week? But the second area that needs to be addressed is the "Right Script-Wrong Player." Mom is obviously feeling a lot of frustration about the "unbalanced ledger" where she perceives dad as getting to do the fun stuff but not having to deal with the To her, this is unfair, and she seems to be pushing on her daughter to "right the wrong" here in order to balance the ledger. This is a good case for the therapist to see if the Mom and Dad would come to the session together in order to better converse about co-parenting, share expectations, and address the ledger.

Exoneration

"Exoneration," although a common Contextual theme and term, can be a big and "dated" word for our younger clients. Therefore, I like to use the terms, "forgiveness," or "let them off the hook," or, "give it up," or, "let it go" when I use this concept in therapy with minor clients and/or their families.

Therapists can use a two-pronged approach to help younger clients understand the concept of, and how to find forgiveness. There is relief in being able to let things go.

1 As mentioned earlier in this chapter, "action" orientation is *key*. When clients are upset or stressed about something, therapists can guide them toward what they can *do* about it.
2 If there is nothing a client can do about something, or the client has *tried* to do something about it and nothing changes, then the client can explore if it's possible to "let go" of it.

Consider the following vignette and how "exoneration" is explored between the therapist and the 14-year-old client, Henry:

Henry: I'm done with them for good [*his teammates from the school soccer team*] and I'm giving them the cold shoulder and I'm not sitting with them at lunch anymore. I won't even look at them or acknowledge them if they say anything to me.

Therapist: Well, I'm sorry to hear that the strategies we talked about to try to resolve things with them haven't seemed to work.

Henry: *Nothing* will work with them. They're just completely self-absorbed, narcissistic, control freaks who don't even realize how stupid they are.

Therapist: Sounds like you're still hanging onto a lot of negative emotion about those guys and how things have been going with them…?

Henry: Yeah, I guess so. It's just really hard to forget what jerks they've been to me and all the other Freshman on the team.

Therapist: Well it seems to me that you have done what you could do to try to change the interactions with them and talk to them about it…and if nothing has changed yet, then maybe it's time to focus on just letting this rest and giving it time to settle?

Henry: But they're still jerks.

Therapist: What would have to happen for you to accept that their behaviors were "jerky" and also accept that you can't change them, and then to let them just be jerks that don't consume a lot of headspace or emotional energy for you?

In subsequent sessions, the therapist helped Henry explore some of the possible reasons the teammates may have acted like they did (insecurity, trying to be "cool" or wanting to create a cohesive upperclassmen "pecking order). Then the therapist brought out his label maker and let Henry choose the tape and font color and created labels for each of the main "jerks" on his soccer team. The therapist had Henry write down each one's name on a separate piece of paper and then slapped a mutually-chosen, brightly colored label on each teammate's sheet:

Tomas—*Anger issues*
Matthew—*Bossy*
Sanjit—*Follower*
Hassan—*Thinks he's cool*
Brendan—*Reckless, self-absorbed, impulsive*

An easier, cheaper alternative for therapists is to just purchase a few sheets of peel-off colored dots (the kind people use to put prices on when they stick them on items at a tag sale) from an office supply store to use instead of the label maker labels.

The therapist was able to help Henry see that all of these "labels" weren't really even about Henry in any way. These were traits that were likely there before Henry came along and would be there whether or not Henry existed in their soccer circle. Letting go of control, frustration over their actions, and focusing more on how Henry wanted to show up around these guys were initial goals. Additionally, the therapist helped Henry expand his thoughts on who he likes and who he would like to become closer friends and how he might be able to make efforts at that.

Case Example

"Willow" is a 12-year-old transgender child who is brought in to therapy for getting in trouble at school when a teacher found their notebook with aggressive drawings and statements in it about self-harm and statements meant to be hurtful to other kids in the school.

A Strategic Therapist's Intervention by "Eon"

Therapist: So Willow, tell me about these drawings and writing that your teacher found in your notebook.

Willow: It was none of her business. She had no right to look at my personal stuff.

Therapist: (*Validating Willow's feelings*) I can understand how that must feel like a violation of your privacy. So can you tell me about what was in there and about the feelings and thoughts you had while writing in your notebook?

Willow: I'm just sick of everyone at my school. They're all mean and critical and rude and are clueless about who I really am, but they still think they have the right to judge me.

At this point, it is clear to Eon that Willow has a "chip on their shoulder" about their perception of being judged or mistreated by classmates. Contextual is a good fit here because it allows Eon to focus on what *they feel entitled to* (respect and understanding from classmates; the teacher respecting Willow's privacy of the notebook) and what *they feel entitled to do in response* to their classmates (write and draw angry, aggressive things about them). Uncovering these and labeling them might be helpful for Eon to introduce to Willow.

Therapist: So you were feeling, what...? Irritated with them? Angry at them? Hurt by them?

Willow: They can't hurt me.

Therapist: Okay, so they don't hurt you, but they make you angry?

Willow: Yup.

Therapist: So when they are critical and rude and mean toward you, you feel like that justifies you thinking about saying hurtful things to them?

Willow: Yeah, then *they'll* understand what it feels like.

Therapist: Okay, so let me get this straight—these kids are mean to you, so if you're mean back to them, then that will "balance" the ledger on both sides and cancel all the mean out?

Willow: I guess.

Therapist: So will that *really* work, Willow? Will everything be fine if you just say something mean back?

Willow: I guess not...

Therapist: So, can we talk about you writing about self-harm? (*After thoroughly assessing for any suicidal ideation and finding not intention or plan, the therapist goes on.*) Can you tell me a bit more about how other kids who are mean to you create a space where you feel like you want to be mean to yourself and stick yourself with pins? I'm not sure that makes sense to me...

Willow: I'm not afraid of pain. I can control it when I do it to myself. It makes me stronger.

Therapist: So does that mean you *don't* feel strong when you aren't sticking yourself with pins? Because I think you're incredibly strong and brave for not only being true to yourself and who you are but also dealing with the meanness from other kids.

Willow: I'm not strong.

Eon continued to explore the concept of destructive entitlements and their impact on Willow's self-image and relationships with others. He coached Willow toward "rejunctive efforts" or how to move toward a place of more mutual trustworthiness. He helped them do this by creating lists of things Willow could *do,* both for themselves, as well as in showing up and managing things around the other kids differently. The therapist used the term, "balance the ledger" on a regular basis to highlight Willow's perception of unfair treatment and what would make the situation seem more fair.

Key Takeaways

Contextual Therapy will always center on a few key concepts when using the model in playful interventions. The following are a few key elements to remember when working from a Contextually-informed lens:

- Contextual therapists highlight the notion that trust and health in relationships emanate from repeated occurrences of ethical and fair interactions. If relationships are *not* trustworthy, entitlement and "debts" start to build up and need to be "paid back."
- Clients keep emotional "ledgers" of unfair actions, and these "unbalanced" ledgers must somehow get "balanced," many times in ways that are destructive to clients and their relationships and often to future generations. This is a key piece for the Contextually-influenced therapist to explore in treatment, and educate clients on.
- This model focuses on the power of how values are passed down through generations, how split and individual loyalties drive people's motivations and behaviors, and the impact of these on not only the here and now but also on future interactions across subsequent generations.

5 Experiential Therapy

Model Background and Key Concepts

Carl Whitaker and Virginia Satir are the names most notable in the Experiential Therapy (e.g., Tuttle, 2003) creation. This model is rooted in the belief that issues come from the suppression of true feelings, lack of understanding, and defense mechanisms "overuse." Feelings and emotional well-being are at the core of this model, as is the notion that by addressing the feelings (inside), the behaviors (outside) improve.

Playful Technique Ideas

Feelings

Since uncovering suppressed emotions is key to this model, therapists need to tend to children's understanding of feelings and their experiences and comfort in expressing them as part of their therapeutic work. There are many ways to do feelings work with minor clients in sessions. The following are a few of my favorites:

- There are a million different free, downloadable, printable "charts" online that have character faces and labeled expressions under each. Conversely, you can make your own by printing out online photos of people making various different facial expressions. For very young clients, it can be a fun discussion to explore what these different people in the photos might be feeling and giving emotion labels to their facial expressions. Additionally, therapists can use these charts regularly to lend a visual gauge for how the child is feeling about certain things discussed in therapy or about events that happened during the week. Feelings "check ins" can be a therapy staple.
- Another (more "hands-on") emotional identification and expression variation to use with very young children is to have them stand up and act out different feelings. For example, the therapist might say, "Show me what you do when you're feeling *angry*." The child might stomp around the room, throwing

DOI: 10.4324/9781003506072-6

pillows, grumbling, and having a snarl on their face. The therapist can then add other things that might also indicate anger like acting out standing in the corner, looking down with a scowl, and arms tightly crossed across the chest.

- Drawing out feelings is a fun exercise to help young clients flesh out their feelings. The therapist can prompt the child to think about what form the feeling "anger" for example would take, what color it would be, and words that describe it. Perhaps the child draws a huge airplane with bright red and orange flames coming out of it and writes words like, "Fiery" or, "Blowing up" or, "Hot" around the plane.

- There are a ton of both therapeutic and mainstream children's books on emotions that are fun to read together with young clients and/or their families. Additionally, there are great movie clips (Like "Inside Out" by Pixar) that are all about emotions and how they show up and are brilliantly acted out as animated characters. A quick You Tube™ search for something similar to, "movie clips on emotions for kids" will yield a zillion hits for a variety of short clips that make great, child-friendly points. For teletherapy clients, watching a clip on a shared screen or keeping a file on your computer with links to clips that you can send clients to do as "homework" are great additions.

- You can order very inexpensively online, tiny, yellow smiley faces with different expressions. These are great to send the child home with as a reminder of a desired emotion. The therapist can also put a smiley face on one sticky note and a frowny face on another sticky note and send them both home with the client to make tally marks on each one for how many times the child felt happy or sad.

"Make the Covert Overt"

Since the notion of uncovering and expressing true emotion is a central element of the Experiential model, the therapist can make efforts to find repressed and hidden things and bring them out when working with children and their families. The following is a clinical vignette with Dad and his two teenage children, Dominic and Gabriela. This is a typical representation of an Experiential therapy session where feelings are being explored, and the therapist attempts to push for the "overt":

Therapist: So, Dad, tell me a bit more about what's going on with the kids.
Dad: Dominic is always rocking the boat at home, pushing the rules, disrespecting everything I say.
Therapist: Go on…
Dad: Yeah, and it just is driving us all crazy, we are just stressed and fighting and it's just not good.
Therapist: When you say it's, "driving us all crazy," who do you mean by "us?"
Dad: I mean me and Gabriela. It makes us crazy.

Therapist: (*Moving over to where Gabriela is sitting and squatting down in front of her*). Gabriela, does Dominic's behavior make you feel crazy?

Gabriela: (*Tentatively.*) Ummm…well not really. I mean, I wish everybody could just get along but I'm not mad at my brother. I get that Dominic is really stressed and I know Dad is stressed out too. But it's fine.

Therapist: Ahhhh, I see. But Gabriela, it's not *really* fine for you, is it? (*Gabriela shrugs*). Are you maybe just a *little bit* mad at Dominic? If he'd just follow the rules, your hope of "everybody getting along" might just happen, huh? (*Gabriela nods.*) So what is it like for you to feel a little bit mad at Dominic for "rocking the boat" at home and a little bit bad for Dad who's stressed by it? And what about Gabriela? Does anyone see how *she* feels in all of this?

When working with preteen and adolescent clients, I generally find the use of a little "friendly jostling" or sarcasm works well to push for covert uncovering. For example, the therapist can ask lightly, "Reallllllllllyyyyyy? Are you sureeeeeee you aren't a teeny, tiny bit hurt by what that girl said to you?" or, "Oh yeah, *of course* it didn't bother you that that girl at school called you a, "privileged, snotty, daddy-issued little brat." I mean, come *on*…why would anybody be hurt or offended by *that* endearing compliment?" This sets the stage for a light, safe, and comfortable disclosure of the possibility of more emotions hidden underneath the surface.

With younger child clients, I often use the "question mark" as a way to push deeper. In my in-person office setting, I used a metal question mark room décor item and would pick it up and set it next to the client after explaining that it symbolized my thought that, "There might be more going on here…?" For teletherapy clients, using the whiteboard to draw a big question mark or putting multiple question marks into the chat are great ways to alert young clients to the possibility of "more feelings under there."

Another clinical "staple" for the Experiential-based, child-friendly therapist is to draw and color a three-leveled picture of the ocean. The surface level is dark blue and the two deeper levels underneath the surface are lighter shades of blue. The therapist can then ask the client, "Are we still talking on the surface level about what's going on at home? (Pointing to the dark blue surface area.) Or is there maybe more, a little deeper here we need to get to?"

Communication Skills/Incongruence

The importance of communication is a central theme in Experiential therapy. Therapists can be helpful in teaching young clients and/or the families better skills in communicating with each other, especially in families where healthy and effective communication was not modeled to them at home.

One lesson to help give young clients in therapy is the importance of having their own voice and speaking for themselves, as opposed to speaking for someone else. The use of a "talking stick" in sessions can set the clear delineation on speaker and listener roles. Just about any object can be used—a pencil, a water bottle, an umbrella, or a decorated, rolled up piece of construction paper. A variation can be to designate a "talking chair" in the therapy room for the speaker to move to when talking. The therapist can also use a small flashlight or a cell phone flashlight to shine on the person speaking. For teletherapy clients, the screen can be angled toward the person speaking. Another idea is to instruct the family to find a safe, lightweight household object (a balled-up sock or wad of tinfoil for example) to toss back and forth to whoever is speaking.

Another important communication lesson is the art of listening and checking in. Much like the old-school game of "telephone" (where a simple message is whispered from person to person down the line until the final person hearing the message speaks it out loud), the message can get distorted in the space between saying it and hearing it. A fun way to practice the importance of good listening skills is to use the practice of "checking in" during sessions.

The therapist can start by modeling this to the client/family from the very first session. Using phrases like, "Hmmm…so tell me if I heard this correctly," or, "I'm not sure if I understand this correctly…" or, "Let me know if I'm way off base here, but I *think* what I heard you say is…" Next, the therapist can introduce the "game" of "feedback" where whenever one person speaks, the therapist asks family members to say what they think they heard the client say. The client then has the opportunity to clarify, refine, or correct the comment based on what the others heard. A fun twist is to have the child client use a thumbs up or thumbs down (emoji on teletherapy sessions) action to report the accuracy of the other family members' feedback.

Another useful tool to use in sessions with minor clients and/or their families is the use of "I statements help clients to speak for *themselves*." If therapists notice a client speaking for someone else or accusing someone of a feeling, they can redirect the client by saying, "Hey, let's try to have you say that again but speaking from *your own* experience, so how about—I feel like…"

"Incongruence" in communication is a concept that Satir really highlighted in her work in building on the Experiential approach. Ideally, when humans speak to one another, their two main levels of communication match each other. For example, one person might say, "I'm fine!" in response to another person asking how they are. If the person says, "I'm fine!" with a smile, warmth, open body energy, and a positive attitude and voice tone, all is good; the verbal message of "I'm fine," matches the non-verbal demeanor. However, sometimes a person might respond, "I'm fine," to the same question, but their body language is closed, their tone terse, a scowl on their face, and perhaps a hint of sarcasm in their voice. In this case, the verbal message of, "I'm fine," doesn't match the non-verbal demeanor and message, thereby leaving younger clients confused and unsettled or worried.

The easiest way to help young clients understand incongruence is by simply role-playing out an example or two like the one offered above. Doing this allows for threefold in the communication work in therapy: (1) Lets clients talk about what they are feeling ("I'm worried that maybe he's *not* fine.") or thinking (ex. "Maybe he's mad at me."), (2) Lets clients brainstorm about what might be going on for the other person, and (3) Lets the clients practice how to ask about the incongruence (ex. "I know you said you're fine, but the way you look and how you said it makes me wonder if you're not totally fine. Is everything okay?")

Role Playing

Role play is a great therapeutic intervention for *any* client, but is especially useful with our younger ones. Role-playing allows for many things:

- "Trying on someone else's shoes" by taking a turn in role-playing another person
- Rehearsing how they might say things to someone else and how they might reply to the various different responses the other person might make
- Use "pretend" skills, which many children are naturally good at
- Adding a fun layer of interaction to traditional talk therapy sessions

A therapist can role play one-on-one with a singular client, but having a sibling or other family members makes the activity all that more interesting and beneficial. For example, having a Mom and her teenage daughter act out how they experience each other talking and relating to them can be both enlightening to the therapist, as well as being a much more experiential event than what traditional verbal descriptions might be.

The role play leaves room for perception changes and a deeper understanding of how the other experiences and feels about their interactions with one another. Additionally, there can even be some space for some humor on occasion. In one family session I was doing with a mother and her 14-year-old daughter, the Mom put on a teenaged voice and flipped her hair and whined, "Ohhhhh my Godddddddd, you are sooooooo attention-gettinggggg," when playing the role of her daughter. The daughter then cracked up and responded with, "No way, you are so off base, Mom! I would never use the word, 'attention getting,' that's *so* something someone *your* age would say!" The Mom laughed too and I redirected to start the role play over using a word the daughter suggested. The Mom laughed again and said, "Ohhhhh my Godddddddd, you are sooooooo thirsty," and the daughter told her that was much more accurate. I offered that it seemed to go much better the second time and that the bonus was that Mom learned a new word from the daughter. The lightness in their interactions was supported by the playful nature of the role play activity.

Sculpting

Sculpting (also sometimes called "psychodrama"), in its most true Experiential form, means literally moving and positioning people into positions and role-playing out (non-verbally) past experiences. It is sort of a creative, active, and dramatic representation of things that have happened to the child. A single client or the entire family can participate in this movement-based activity. The client and/or family can act out past events and feelings by positioning themselves or others. For example, if there was a family fight that a six-year-old client ("Rafaela") is describing in session, the therapist may instruct her to move and position her family members as she sees fit. She might have her Dad stand up on the couch beating his chest and roaring like a lion, while she and her brother are curled up in a fetal position under the table, and her Mom is sitting cross-legged on the floor laughing at Dad.

The therapist is free to intervene at times, asking questions or offering guidance, ideas, or instruction. If the session contains more than one client, family members can take turns being the "sculptor" and the members can discuss afterward what some of the differences were in perception, how things could go differently next time, and how they felt about doing the activity. Generally, young clients love "being the boss" as the sculptor, and enjoy participating in fun, active movement things in therapy.

Puppet Interviews

This therapeutic technique was a favorite of Virginia Satir and can be seen in various different forms across a multitude of child sessions today. The use of puppets, dolls, or figurines lends itself so well to the typical playful ways therapists can engage children in treatment. At the same time, the information gleaned by the therapist from observing the puppet activities is vital to understanding family dynamics.

Child clients and/or their family members can select a puppet, doll, or other figurine or stuffed animal to represent themselves and/or their various family members. Clients can include puppets to represent other pertinent people in their lives like teachers, babysitters, or peers that may play a part in what is going on in the children's lives. The client and/or family members are then asked to act out or tell a little story about their family or issues that have been going on through their puppets. Conversely, different family members can have conversations with one another through their puppets. This technique can be used as a way to create a symbolic representation of the actual issues, and clients can experience better comfort and safety in communicating about them through their puppets.

For the therapist, the playful and therapeutic activity of puppet interviews can reveal helpful information, like the etiology of conflicts, dysfunctional patterns of communication or behavior, feelings, or where things like alliance, coalitions, or triangulation might exist.

Variations of puppet interviews can include simple dollhouse play where the child labels the dolls that live in the house as family members and the therapist can simply observe the interactions between the dolls or ask the child questions about the interactions. Likewise, the therapist can ask the child to act out bedtime, for example, using the family member dolls and the rooms in the house.

Another alternative to the puppet interviews is to engage the child in the artistic creation of decorated face circles for each family member. The faces can be ordered in bulk as blank faces, printed off of the many available on sites online, or just have the child cut out circles on copier paper. Specialty copier paper comes in a variety of shades that might be better suited for children to select the paper color that best matches their own skin color. The child can draw on the faces, or the therapist can order online stickers that offer a variety of color, shape, and size of things like eyes, mustaches, noses, and mouths. This variation is particularly fitting for use with teletherapy clients who can create their own faces at home during the session. Popsicle sticks, or the larger tongue depressor sticks can be purchased online or at craft stores.

"Head and Heart" Game

"Head and Heart" is a game I play with younger clients to help them understand the Experiential concept of needing to "get out of our heads, and into our emotions." I use a laminated hand-drawn red heart cut out, and a gray brain-shaped cutout for this activity. When a client is speaking from their "head" (ex: "My little sister always gets her way because she just tattles on me and whines to Mom and Mon just believes her and gives in to whatever my sister wants. One time, she even made me give the last mini-bag of cookies to my sister because she lied to Mom and told her I had already eaten two other bags of them"), I might place the heart cutout on their lap and say, "Good job speaking from your head, but now I want to hear you speaking from your heart." The child may then respond, "I'm so mad at my sister! I feel bad because I think Mom likes her best and I feel like I'm a bad kid because I'm always getting in trouble."

Another variation is to leave the two cutouts next to the client and ask them to choose which one to hold as they are saying different things. The therapist can always use modeling to give examples of what things we can say that are "heart" things and which ones are more "mind" things. There are many different replicas of brains and hearts available to buy online as well--from stickers to figurines, to little wind-up toys. However, oftentimes young clients enjoy the process of creating or using hand-crafted artistic manipulatives in the session with the therapist, and this way the therapist can choose to send home some of these tools so that the child will be more likely to remember to utilize them outside of sessions.

Case Example

The therapist, "Lucinda," is working with four-year-old Laiba and her six-year-old brother, Hassan. The kids were referred to therapy by their guardian (their maternal grandmother) after both of their parents were killed in violence in their home country. The children were taken to the US two years prior to live with the grandmother who lived there. Laiba had been asked to leave her preschool due to stealing things and for biting other children, and Hassan was identified in first grade as "at-risk" due to problems with focusing, not listening, and falling behind academically. The children were also seeing a pediatric trauma specialist certified in play therapy once a week.

An Experiential Therapist's Intervention by "Lucinda"

Therapist: So, last week grandma was telling us about all the sad and bad things that have happened to your family and I wondered if you might play a game with me today that will help me understand how you *feel* about all of those things. (*The therapist stretches out the plastic mat from the popular Twister™ game with the big colored dots all over it.*)

Hassan: I wanna play it! (*Jumping around on the mat.*)

Therapist: Okay, so here is how it goes. I'm going to write a feeling on a sticky note and stick it on one of the circles on the mat. I'm going to choose the feeling of 'sad.' Can one of you come help me pick which color sticky note we should pick for 'sad?'

Laiba: Blue!

Therapist: Why blue, Laiba?

Laiba: Because tears are blue in picture books when someone cries. And we cry from our eyes, and mine are blue.

Therapist: Perfect! (*Writes, "BLUE" on the sticky note and sticks it inside a yellow circle.*) Now, everyone in the room, who has ever felt sad, put a foot or a hand in the sad circle when I say 'go!' Go! (*The kids both go to the circle and put a foot in it.*)

Therapist: Now, while your feet are on the sad circle, I want you to yell out one thing that makes you feel sad.

Hassan: School!

Laiba: Mean kids!

Therapist: Hmmmmm…anything else that makes you sad?

Hassan: When we have fish for dinner!

Laiba: Not having a mommy or daddy.

Therapist: Those are lots of sad things. Good job. Can you both show me the faces you make when you feel sad? (*Kids make sad faces, and Laiba balls up her fists, rubs them against her eyes, and makes fake crying sounds.*) Oh good, Laiba! I forgot about what *sounds* we make when we are sad. Okay, so on the count of three, I want you both to make sad faces, make sad sounds, and make sad body movements, okay? One...two...three!

Therapist: Now, can you come sit over here with me for a minute, Laiba? I want you to choose one of these puppets that you think is most like you. (*Laiba chooses a lion with a fluffy mane.*) Why did you choose the lion, Laiba?

Laiba: Because it roars and scares everybody.

Therapist: Do you "roar" and scare anybody, Laiba? (*Laiba nods.*)

Therapist: Okay, Hassan, your turn—come pick a puppet that best suits YOU. (*Hassan chooses a kangaroo.*) Why did you choose the kangaroo, Hassan?

Hassan: Because they can jump away fast if they want to.

Therapist: Do you ever feel like you want to jump away fast?

Hassan: Yes! Everyday. I hate school. I want to kangaroo away from school! (*Hassan jumps around the room like a kangaroo.*)

Therapist: Okay, I have another feelings game. I'm going to ask "Laiba the lion" and Hassan the kangaroo" to talk to each other about something sad. And if it's okay, I might want to whisper a question or idea into the lion or the kangaroo's ear. Let's sit across from each other on the 'sad spot' and I can't wait to hear what the lion and kangaroo are going to tell us!

Lucinda continued to explore the concept of sadness with the kids in subsequent sessions, with a strong focus on exploring the *feeling* of sadness, rather than on the events that were sad. Additionally, Lucinda's placement of the blue 'sad' sticky on the yellow Twister™ circle was intentional. This was because she later used the contrasting colors to label the yellow as the feeling of "happy" and began the exploration of whether "happy" and "sad" could both exist together and take turns when they show up. She spent some time with the kids doing the same feelings activities with the "happy" as she had done with the "sad" and helping the children toward actions that made them feel happy or sad.

Key Takeaways

Experiential Therapy will always center on a few key concepts when using the model in playful interventions. The following are a few key elements to remember when working from an experientially-informed lens:

- Feelings and emotional well-being are at the core of this model. Therefore, Experientially-guided therapists should strive to challenge clients to "go deeper" and delve into the feelings that exist behind the thoughts and actions of themselves and of others when they come up in the therapy room.
- Experiential therapists adhere to the notion that the feelings (inside) are the key to the symptomatic behaviors (outside) improving. Embracing this, therapists should be mindful of not focusing on the things a client is doing or saying, but rather on what the client is *feeling*.
- As one of the most organically playful models of therapy, Experiential therapists have a wide range of interventions to lean on for hands-on, emotional work. Things like puppet interviews and role play are great tools for use in kid client treatment.

6 Narrative Therapy

Model Background and Key Concepts

Michael White, David Epston, Jill Freedman, and Gene Combs are the familiar names associated with the Narrative Therapy (White & Epston, 1990) model. One basic tenet of the model includes the notion that there is no one true "reality," but rather that "reality" is both socially constructed and shaped by the language used to describe it. Another central idea is that people tell "stories" (or "narratives") that define things and that these stories shape their ideas, perceptions, and actions. These stories are often based on the messages we receive from society and our families of origin.

Playful Technique Ideas

Stories/Narratives

One of the most powerful principles of Narrative therapy is the idea of how people's reality is based on the stories they create. In this model, they call these stories "narratives." Working through the mode of storytelling is an enjoyable and effective way to use therapy with child clients.

The first step for using storytelling as a modality for treatment is in the language therapists use with clients. For example, things like, "Wow! That's a really difficult story for me to hear," or, "So that's the story in a nutshell of how you explain how your brother is treating you," or, "So that's a lot of history that's gone on between you and your brother...what's the story you think he tells about why you guys haven't been getting along?" Doing this introduces and normalizes the concept that we *all* create stories or narratives from our experiences. Additionally, using this method, therapists can begin to expose children to the idea of how each of our own narratives links to so many other things like the choices we make, how we view others, or our behaviors. Adding this layer of understanding to interpersonal communication and relations can help children develop a broader view of the relationships and interactions that children have with others.

DOI: 10.4324/9781003506072-7

After introducing and using the concept of stories or narratives on a regular basis with younger clients, therapists can become more bold about how they "challenge" kids on their narratives. For example, one might choose to say,

> So Maria, do you think your mom *really* hates you, or is that the story you've created for yourself? Do you think that maybe another possible narrative here is that mom is frustrated with not being able to make you understand that she is concerned and worried about some of your choices and wants to keep you safe? And maybe she is trying to control your safety in the best way she know how and it doesn't always come across that way? Is that another possible story?

This allows therapists to not "choose sides" or discount the child's "truth," but rather to offer up another possibility. Opening up the space for a narrative a little bit different than their own may help in dispelling some inaccuracies or decreasing some of the anger or animosity in a gentle way. Additionally, this allows therapists to maintain a therapeutic alliance with the child.

Multiple "Truths"

A related concept to the stories and narratives above is the idea that there is no singular "truth," but that everybody creates their own based on things like perceptions, internalized meaning from experiences, personal biases, belief systems, etc. Eliminating the idea that there is one truth or an absolute right or wrong in how things are seen by individuals can help children learn acceptance, understanding, and tolerance in their interactions with others.

One of my favorite therapeutic activities to use with younger children is the retelling of whatever children's story or fairytale they are familiar with. I have found this activity to be actually quite enjoyable and meaningful for adults/parents who have been present for this as well. Having props or animals or figurines to act out the story is a great hands-on addition to the activity.

One tale that has worked well for therapists using this activity is the classic story of "Cinderella." Please note that if therapists have any concerns about the traditional stereotypes included in this story (e.g., the demure main character who is prized for her physical attractiveness and sweet demeanor), there are countless other choices of stories to use for this activity. Additionally, therapists can personalize the story they choose to best fit the cultural, socioeconomic, ethnic, or family member makeup specifics of any given client.

The first step is a simple retelling of the story of Cinderella. This is where therapists can adhere to the simplest template of the story, thereby avoiding any details that are stereotypical or contain unwanted messaging. After summarizing the story, therapists can ask the child to consider the views of a few of the main characters—Cinderella, the step-sisters, the step mother, the Prince, and

Cinderella's father. The therapist can start off by offering an example of one of the following:

Cinderella: I'm so sad, I just lost my mother and wish that my new step mother could love me. I've never had siblings and I had so hoped that my new sisters and I would have fun together and enjoy getting to know each other—why are they so mean to me? I try to be nice and help out whenever I can but I just don't seem to be good enough...

The Step-Sisters: Why did the mother marry that girl's father? He's never here and never helps out and mama has to do all the work so Cinderella should do the fair share for both of them. Cinderella isolates herself and is aloof and not very friendly. We have so much to offer her here, we saved her and she's ungrateful and always goes off to be alone. She wants to steal our boyfriends, it's so obvious how innocent and sweet she acts, but it's all manipulation...

The Step Mother: This girl's father gives us money and support, but I'm stuck having to care for another child, another mouth to feed. She has an instant family and should help out around here to earn her keep. My daughters work hard to get what they want and Cinderella breezes in here selfishly, trying to take things she hasn't worked for or earned, and steal them from my daughters...

The Prince: Fortune and fame do not buy me happiness. These women around here only want me for my money. I am looking for a partner, someone with substance and kindness and a heart that cares about others. Who is this new young woman in town? She exudes such a genuine kind and caring energy. She is earnest and hardworking. I'd like to get to know her better...

Cinderella's Father: My poor daughter! Lost her mother and I'm often not there for her, I don't know how to fill the void of a mother to her. I have found a step-mother and step-sisters to take her in, love her, and care for in ways I cannot do. This wonderful woman is willing to embrace Cinderella and love and care for her like her own. This is a perfect match!

From here, there are many ways the therapist can use the Cinderella activity. For example, asking about what the different value systems each character has (a.k.a., what's important to them), what things might have happened to each character that contributed to their narrative, how could any two of the characters talk to each other in a way that would yield better understanding of each other, etc.

Additionally, therapists can use a follow-up of the activity using real-life "characters" of people in the client's life that contribute to, sustain, or are part of the problem to open up the possibilities of meaning and intention. For example, therapists might ask child clients to tell a story about how mom, grandma, and older brother would explain and feel about a recent family argument.

For an online therapy adaptation, therapists can find numerous children's fairytales or summaries of stories to look at together online, many with beautiful artistic embellishments. There is audio of many classic fairytales online. Almost any children's TV show clip can be found (for example, on YouTube™) online that therapists and children can watch together and use as a jumping off point for the discussions provided above.

Deconstructing

"Deconstruction" can sometimes be called "unpacking." Either term resonates well with younger clients when using them as playful interventions. For deconstruction, blocks or Legos™ are perfect for use. For younger clients, it's easy to explain the way we build up things by stacking the blocks up high, and then how we deconstruct them by knocking them down. This is part one. For older kids, the therapist can write things on a small pile of sticky notes and then pull each one apart, ripping up (or otherwise destroying) the ones the therapist and client deem not entirely true.

For part two, the therapist can offer examples of how we build things up. For instance, let's take 14-year-old "Freddie," who comes to therapy for being aggressive and starting fights at school. The therapist might ask Freddie to give ideas about what his teachers and classmates think about him. Freddie responds with a list of descriptors that includes, "Bad-ass, dumb, troublemaker, rude." The therapist writes these words down, one on each of four sticky notes. Then the therapist discusses each one thoroughly, deconstructing them and looking for evidence that they might not be entirely true. Consider the following vignette between the therapist and Freddie:

Therapist: So you had me write down "dumb" on one of these sticky notes about how your teachers and classmates think about you. Do you think you're "dumb?"

Freddie: Kinda, yeah. I mean I fail a lot of tests and don't do my homework.

Therapist: Okay, but failing tests and not doing homework just means you're probably not studying or doing assignments and that's why you get bad grades, right? But that doesn't necessarily mean you're dumb...

Freddie: I guess.

Therapist: So if I told you I was gonna give you $100 if you studied for an English test and passed it, could you do it?

Freddie: (*Laughs.*) Yeh. Probably. For a hundred bucks I could...

Therapist: (*Ripping up the sticky note with "dumb" on it and tossing it in the garbage can.*) Okay, so "dumb" is not the right word here. Let's replace "dumb" with a better fitting word, what do you think?

Freddie: Lazy.

Therapist: Are you *sure* it's lazy? Think about it for a minute...

Freddie: Okay, it's like I just don't ever feel like doing the homework or studying.

Therapist: (*Writing on a new sticky note.*) Okay, I think I've got the right word. "Unmotivated."

Freddie: Yeh!

For "unpacking" therapists can help children draw an empty suitcase and decide what things they will need to put inside it for a trip. If they will be traveling to a beach for example, they will need to pack a swimsuit, flip flops, tee-shirts, sunscreen, goggles, a float, etc. The therapist can then add a few items like snow boots, a winter hat, ice skates, a mug of hot cocoa to the drawing. Consider the vignette below between the therapist and seven-year-old Emma:

Emma: That's silly! Why did you draw boots and ice skates for a vacation to the *beach?*

Therapist: Oh, did I?! That *is* silly, isn't it?

Emma: We don't need snow boots at the beach! And a mug of hot cocoa would spill all over everything and ruin all your clothes.

Therapist: You're right. Maybe we should *unpack* everything and start over?

Emma: Okay.

Therapist: (*Pointing to one item in the suitcase at a time*). Do we need a swimsuit, thumbs up or thumbs down?

Emma: (*Nods and gives the thumbs-up sign.*)

Therapist: Do we need goggles? Is there a pool on your vacation at the beach?

Emma: No, just a cottage on the ocean.

Therapist: Okay, so do you use goggles when you swim in the ocean or only when you swim in a pool?

Emma: Just in the pool.

Therapist: Okay, so looks like we can unpack the goggles! (*Therapist crosses out the goggles with a red marker.*) Now let's cross out the other easy ones we don't need—you said hot cocoa would spill and ruin the clothes, right? So let's cross that one out.

Emma: And the boots and the hat and the ice skates!

Therapist: So Emma, I was thinking about how the issues you came here for, about self-esteem and being angry at yourself might also be things we can talk about unpacking.

Emma: How do you mean?

Therapist: Well, let's talk about a typical school day in second grade, okay? Pretend we have a suitcase for the school day. (*Therapist draws a big, open, empty two-sided suitcase on a piece of paper.*) So, shall we put pens and pencils in it?

Emma: (*Laughs.*) Of course!

Therapist: How about a water bottle? (*Emma nods.*) And your notebook and reading glasses? (*Emma gives the thumbs-up.*) Okay, now about, "Nobody likes me," should *that* get packed to bring to school?

Emma: (*Looking sad.*) The "nobody likes me" thoughts *always* come with me.

Therapist: Okay, but what about if we left it at home one day? I don't think you really need to be dragging the "nobody likes me" thought around all day—that's not very fun when you are trying to learn or eat lunch or play at recess, is it? So do you really think *nobody* likes you? (*Emma nods.*) Well how about the teacher? And your bus driver. Do *they* like you?

Emma: I guess so.

Therapist: So who doesn't like you, Emma?

Emma: Shelby, Arianna, and Ming. They never let me play with them.

Therapist: Hmmmmm, so they never let you *play* with them, but we don't know why they don't? (*Emma shakes her head.*) So we're not sure if they don't like you. But we are pretty sure they don't invite you to play with them, right? (*Emma nods.*) So I think we need to cross out the "nobody likes me" thought and try leaving at home this week because we know a few people who *do* like you at school, and we are not sure about the ones who don't let you play with them.

The therapist then continued on with brainstorming ways that Emma might try to do things differently at school to increase the chances the girls would let her play with them *or* how Emma could try to make friends with other kids in her class other than the three who wouldn't let her play with them. The scenario describes a playful way for the therapist help Emma to understand how one "message" from her social group began Emma building a narrative about nobody liking her that became incredibly big and powerful.

Unique Outcomes

"Unique Outcomes" are exceptions to what clients' stories or narratives would make them believe would happen. In short, unique outcomes are when the expected thing (like feeling angry) *doesn't* happen. This is very similar to the notion of "exceptions" that the Solution Focused model looks for in times when the "problem" *isn't* occurring. Especially with kids and parents, it can be easy for them to focus on the "bad" things or the problems and forget to notice the times when the problem *isn't* there. Changing problematic patterns doesn't always have to focus on the problems themselves. Often, it is easier to focus on what's going on when the problem *isn't* there and figure out how to do more of *that* so that it becomes the new norm and crowds out the old problematic patterns.

The easiest way to help introduce younger clients to this concept is simply with the *language*. Consider the following vignette between the therapist and 12-year-old Kiki:

Therapist: Wow, so that is a *LOT* of times that your friend Melanie "stood you up." Sounds like something has changed in your relationship with her.

Kiki: Yeah. We used to *always* hang out, text each other every day, do something like every weekend.

Therapist: So what happens now?

Kiki: She doesn't really text me and never asks me to do anything on the weekends.

Therapist: Is there a reason she might not be up for going out lately? Depressed? Just wanting to chill at home? Something going on that you don't know about?

Kiki: Maybe, but I doubt it. I see her post stuff on social media and she's out and looks like she's having a good time.

Therapist: Are there times when she *does* reach out to you?

Kiki: Sometimes she does. But not often.

Therapist: So what's different about those times when she *does* reach out?

From this point, the therapist can work with Kiki to figure out what's different and how to do more of it. In this case, Kiki shared that when she reached out first to her friend, *and* if they shared some positive or genuine communication, it seemed like her friend was more receptive to keeping the conversation going. From here, the therapist suggested that Kiki think about finding ways to communicate more deeply about things and how she was feeling to her friend. In this vignette, the unique outcomes (what to do *more* of that seemed to be present when the problem *wasn't* happening) were the focus, rather than on the problem (the friend continuing to blow Kiki off).

Externalization

The concept of externalization is an important concept for use in playful interventions with young clients. According to Narrative Therapy, the *problem* is the problem—the *person* is not the problem. Therefore, therapists want clients to understand that the problem lies *outside* of them, rather than *inside*, as part of them. Externalizing is also helpful when working with families, as it decreases the chances of families criticizing or ascribing responsibility toward individual members for the problem, but rather being able to collectively tackle the (external) problem together. This allows for a "same team" mentality, rather than for a "blame game" one. The following are some creative and playful examples of how to externalize problems when working with kid clients and/or their families.

One of the easiest ways to introduce young clients to the concept of externalization is for the therapist to put the word "the" in front of whatever issue or problem is being discussed. For example, if a ten-year-old is getting in trouble for frequently getting angry at a sibling, the therapist can say, "So, tell me about when ___*the*___ anger shows up." This subtlety separates *the* anger from the child. Additionally, if a child says something like, "I'm angry all the time," the therapist can reframe and state back to the child, "It sounds like ___*the*___ anger has been hanging around and bugging you lately, making your life a little tough, huh?"

Another fun intervention to use with kid clients is to create a "monster" that represents the problem or issue (e.g., "anger") being worked on. First, therapists should assess the client to be sure that there are no fears of monsters. Then, the child can draw and color a picture of a monster on a piece of paper. The therapist can coach child clients to choose colors they feel best to represent their feelings about the "monster." They can write words around it such as, "yelling," or, "scary," or, "hot."

This is an activity that externalizes the problem from the client and makes it a "monster" outside of them. The therapist can ask the client and/or family members at the beginning of each week how the "anger monster" has been showing up. Using scaling questions from a previous (Solution Focused) chapter is a good way for the client and/or family members to rate the "monster's" behavior from 1 to 10. This helps everyone to gauge how prominent the "monster" has been, thereby tracking progress toward the intended goal (e.g., reduced anger).

An additional, playful twist on the externalizing monster intervention is to write "Anger Monster" on a sticky note. Then, when the problem of it is very big (like at the beginning of therapy), the therapist can stick the note on the wall of the office way above the child's head. The therapist can explain that the "monster" seems out of reach to the child because it is too big and too strong. Each week the therapist can help the client strategize about what things could maybe make the "monster" smaller. As the anger decreases over treatment, the therapist moves the sticky note down lower until it is even with the child's eye level. Now the two are "even."

When the anger problem has gone away, the child can remove the sticky and "dispose" of it. Some popular ideas are to rip it up and put it in the garbage, tear it into tiny pieces and vacuum them up, bury the shredded sticky outside somewhere, or color all over it with black marker. One of my favorite disposal methods is to add the pieces of the ripped-up sticky with ripped-up pieces of colored construction paper and stuff them all in a half-full bottle of water. The bottle sits in the therapist's office until the next session. Over time, the colors bleed and tint the water, the print on the sticky becomes illegible, and the child can take the bottle home to shake whenever thoughts of anger creep in.

For in-person therapy, a dollhouse or stuffed animals can be used to act our scenes from the client's family or social interactions, making the dolls or animals the *characters* in the scenes, rather than the actual client, friends, or family members. The therapist can allow the client(s) to choose which dolls or animals will represent the family members and the roles they each take on.

Many of the aforementioned ideas can be adapted for remote sessions. Most families will have a plastic bottle, water, markers, colored paper, and sticky notes somewhere in the house, and most children can find animals or figurines in their homes as well. In the rare case that there are no figurines or animals in the home, the child can use any common household objects to represent the members of their family or social group.

Reauthoring

"Reauthoring" is an exciting idea to share with clients and their families. Clients can take their story or narrative and change it going forward, or looking back, rewriting it to a healthier one that includes more empowerment, control, and healthy attitude. For example, therapists can start by asking child clients (when they are sharing an upsetting situation), "Okay, so if you could do it over, how would you do it differently?"

Another great use of reauthoring is in using the example of storytelling with younger clients. The therapist and client can read a short children's book together (or online for remote sessions) and then talk about how the story could have been different if the various characters chose to do other things. It's important to note for children that stories don't really end, but continue to evolve and carry into new chapters, and that the child can have some choice in how the stories go.

My favorite intervention to use with younger clients and/or their families is what I call the "story bag." The purpose of the story is twofold. First, it allows the child to understand how each piece of the story impacts the next piece and how there is always another choice that follows. The second is so that the therapist maintains a hand in controlling the direction of the story activity so that it stays pertinent to the therapeutic goals and the specific occurrences in the child's life. In the final case example below, "Rosalita" will use a Narrative approach to working with seven-year-old "Ricky," and demonstrate the use of the "story bag" intervention.

Case Example

Seven-year-old Ricky is brought to therapy by his grandmother who has recently become his guardian after Ricky's father killed his mother and himself in a murder-suicide. Ricky has been expressing a lot of anger toward his grandmother and other kids at school. Additionally, Ricky has been telling people that he now believes that just everybody is going to die soon.

A Narrative Therapist's Intervention by "Rosalita"

Therapist: Hi, Ricky! My name is Rosalita. I understand that you're here to talk about some things that have happened in your family.

Ricky: Yeah. My dad shot my mother. And himself. And now I live with my grandma.

Therapist: Wow. Grandma also told me that you've been talking a lot about everybody dying soon. Tell me about that...

Ricky: Well, my grandpa died last year, and my teacher from kindergarten had cancer and died, and my baby brother died the day after he was born. And my parents. And the man who lives next door. Either me or my grandma is next.

Therapist: So that's what you think, huh?

Ricky: Yup. Pretty sure.

Therapist: How do you feel when you think about that?

Ricky: Mad.

Therapist: I bet. I can see that. How about scared? Do you feel scared when you think about that?

Ricky: Kinda. But not really.

Therapist: So one story we could tell is that because so many people have died around you, chances are that you and grandma are next. (*Ricky nods.*) But could there be another story here?

Ricky: Like what?

Therapist: Well, that all those deaths were terrible and too many to happen in one young person's life since you've only been here for seven years! Could that be true?

Ricky: I guess that's true.

Therapist: Could it also be true that you have used up a whole lot of the deaths that will happen in your life and that there won't be any more for a very long time?

Ricky: (*Looking very surprised at this thought.*) I don't know...

Therapist: I'd love to play the "story bag" game with you—do you want to play? (*Ricky nods.*) So I have this cloth bag full of a bunch of little objects, see? (*Therapist lets Ricky peek into the top of the bag.*) So the way it works is that we are going to tell a story together and each add pieces to it as we take turns pulling an object from inside the bag. Got it? (*Ricky nods.*) Okay, I'll go first to show you how we play. (*Therapist reaches in and pulls out a big, red bullseye glass marble with red and blue swirls.*) So once upon a time, there was a big roly-poly marble who wanted to find a friend. Now it's your turn, Ricky.

Ricky: (*Pulls a tiny white dog figurine from the bag.*) Then Mr. Marble met a dog friend and he was happy. But then he was sad because he knew the dog would run away.

Therapist: (*Pulling out a pliable yellow sun-shaped eraser from the bag*). But then Mr. Marble remembered that whenever the sun came out, and even on a rainy day, the sun would always come out again on another day, the dog would come back to play. So then he was happy again.

This game was something Rosalita used on several occasions with Ricky to demonstrate openings for where new outcomes could turn up, even when Ricky was storying that there would be one fixed outcome. Rosalita interspersed the "story bag" activity with externalizing the thoughts of death and loss and tracking them to see how they could make them settle down a bit and leave Ricky alone sometimes.

The "story bag" intervention works just as well with teletherapy. In the remote session case, the therapist would just pull an object out for the client and hold it up to the screen so they could see what prompt they got for continuing the story.

Key Takeaways

Narrative Therapy will always center on a few key concepts when using the model in playful interventions. The following are a few key elements to remember when working from a Narratively-informed lens:

- One basic tenet of the model includes the notion that there is no one true "reality," but rather that "reality" is both socially constructed and shaped by the language used to describe it. This is a key concept for Narratively-based therapists to use when deciding on language to use in sessions, and how to help clients understand the multiplicity of "valid" views. It is also important for therapists to remember that their own view of the client/family is biased and not "truth."
- Another central idea in Narrative work is that people tell "stories" (or "narratives") that define things and that these stories shape their ideas, perceptions, and actions. These stories are often based on the messages they receive from society and our families of origin. Helping kid clients and/or their families understand the power of these stories and messages is paramount in treatment.
- Narrative Therapy lends itself to many playful ways for child clients to understand important concepts. The use of storytelling, reauthoring, and externalizing problems are fun and easy to use with younger clients.

7   Solution Focused Brief Therapy (SFBT or SFT)

Model Background and Key Concepts

The SFBT or SFT model of therapy (e.g., de Shazer, 1982) was founded by Insoo Kim Berg and Steve de Shazer. The model is known for its focus on solution building, instead of on problem saturation in therapy. There are many techniques they created to do this, and most are incredibly suitable for young client work. Other highlights of the model are the focus on the present and future instead of on the past, that the "problem" is *not* occurring *all* the time, and that we only need a *small* change in order for the "snowball effect" to organically create bigger changes.

Playful Technique Ideas

The Miracle Question

In traditional SFT language, the Miracle Question is some variation of this: "Let's say you went home tonight and went to sleep and when you woke up, a miracle had happened. Tell me what would have changed?" This question prompts clients toward the place where the problems are gone and has them talk about what that place is like. Not only is there a positive, more solution-focused emphasis here, but the responses to the Miracle Question swiftly lay out goals for the client. Consider the following with 11-year-old Lucas:

Therapist: So, Lucas…I want to ask you an interesting question to help me understand your situation a little better. If you left our session today and went home, went to bed, and woke up the next morning and a miracle had happened, what would have changed?

Lucas: I'd be an only child and not have an annoying little brother who gets away with everything and gets all Mom's attention!

Therapist: Hmmm…okay, and what else?

Lucas: This kid in my class, Trey, would be nice to me.

DOI: 10.4324/9781003506072-8

Therapist: Okay…

Lucas: Mom would let me eat ice cream for every meal.

Therapist: (*Laughs.*) Okay, so those would be some big miracles, huh? So Lucas, I took some notes on your miracles so I could list some things that we can work on in sessions. Wanna hear them?

Lucas: Sure!

Therapist: Okay, the first miracle would be you woke up an only child without an annoying little brother who got away with everything and took all Mom's attention, right? (*Lucas nods.*) So I wrote down that one goal for us to work on is to figure out how to be less annoyed by your brother, have more fairness in things at home with what you two are allowed to do, and maybe to get a little bit more time one-on-one with Mom. What do you think?

Lucas: HA! Yeah, right, well if all THAT happened it would be a miracle for sure!

Therapist: Okay, we can move on to miracle number two now, but first, I want to let you know that I think that last miracle, the one about ice cream for every meal, I don't think I'm going to be able to help you too much with *that* one. I'm thinking *that* one's going to be a real stretch to get Mom to allow, don't you? (*Laughter.*)

With younger clients, I often rename the miracle question as the "magic wand question." For an extra fun touch, you can use an item from your office (or from the child's home if it is teletherapy) to represent the "magic wand." You can order all sorts of magic wands for kids online, or you can make one in session by using a paper towel tube, tape, and construction paper. My child clients' favorite wand was a tiny glow in the dark one I found in some old Barbie stuff that one of my daughters had. Turning out the office lights (for children who are not uncomfortable or fearful of the dark) to wave the glowing magic wand was the highlight of weekly sessions for many of my kid clients. Craft stores have glow-in-the-dark paint that therapists can use to paint a hand-crafted magic wand as well.

Exceptions

Since SFT believes that the problem is *not* always happening, therapists will look for "exceptions" or times when the problem *isn't* happening. It is very common for younger clients to see the world in absolutes. For example, kids will often say things like, "My mom _never_ lets me stay up late" or, "John _always_ gets to play the game at school."

One of my favorite ways to help young clients to begin to understand the concept of "exceptions" is to brainstorm about what other words might be better substituted for the common absolutes of "always' and "never." If you need help, just use a search engine to look for "always" antonyms. For example, instead of using "always," the following are some better alternatives:

- A lot of the time
- Mostly
- Consistently
- Regularly
- Often
- Constantly
- Almost always

Using these alternate words creates the assumption that there are in fact, at least *sometimes* when the problem doesn't occur. It's helpful to have young clients begin to understand that if even *once* the problem doesn't happen, then *maybe* we can figure out how to have it happen less. This is a good place to ground SFT treatment on for both young clients, as well their parents or guardians who can also benefit from understanding that problems aren't happening *all* of the time. This is especially true when it seems that they are ignoring the more positive behaviors that their children might be displaying along with the poor ones.

Another playful way to help clients with understanding exceptions is to regularly insert, "Except...?" when a child is telling an "always" or "never" story. The following example is how one therapist opened up this door for his client, Treyvon:

Treyvon: This kid at school is *whack*. He's always being like up in the teacher's face *every* time she asks us to do anything. And he's always up in my face too, trying to talk crazy and threaten me.

Therapist: Wow. That sounds pretty stressful.

Treyvon: Yeah. I'm over it. Can't deal with his attitude.

Therapist: (*After assessing for any threat or intention of harm to the other kid from the client.*) Okay, so tell me about a time when the kid *wasn't* all up someone's face.

Treyvon: No man, he's *always* up in somebody's face...

Therapist: Except...?

Treyvon: Except what?

Therapist: So he's all up in somebody's face *except* when...there must be a time when he minds his own business?

Treyvon: Well yeah, when he's stuffing his face with food at lunch or taking a leak maybe.

Therapist: Okay, so what might be different about the times he *isn't* up in people's faces? Is there anything we can think of that might increase the chances he'll mind his own business more often? What's different about when he's eating or going to the bathroom?

Treyvon: Nobody's asking him to do nothing.

Therapist: Aha! You might have something there. So when other people leave him alone and don't ask him to do anything, he minds his own business?

Scaling Questions

Scaling questions are especially great for kid clients, especially the younger ones. Scaling questions simply mean that the we use a number system (0–10 or 1–10) to help kids respond to questions we ask. This allows a more globally understood way of measuring, as opposed to finding just the right combination of words to accurately describe what a client is thinking. For example, instead of asking a child, "How are you feeling today?" (which might elicit a general, "okay," response), the therapist might ask, "On a scale of 1–10, with 1 being the lowest, saddest place, and 10 being the best day of your life happy place, how are you feeling today?" This allows the language and "fleshing out" of the number the child gives to come secondarily, only *after* the therapist gets an immediate number than can help gaugewhere the child is coming into session.

Another benefit of using scaling questions is that it is easier to gauge progress in *tiny* increments, while still being able to note the change. The following vignette with a therapist, 13-year-old Marcus, and his Mom demonstrates how scaling in tiny increments can be used:

Therapist: Okay, so let's talk about how the week went. Marcus, on a scale of 0–10, with a "0" meaning no problems at all this week, it was an awesome week, and a "10" meaning it was a terrible week, maybe the worst ever, how would you rate the last week?

Marcus: Ummm… maybe a 4.

Therapist: Okay, tell me a bit about why the week was a '4.'

Marcus: Because my Mom still nagged me a lot, shut off my video game right in the middle of a high score *twice*, and yelled at me about everything, even though she promised she wouldn't.

Therapist: Okay, so Mom, what number rating would you give the last week on how things went?

Mom: I'd agree with Marcus. A solid '4.'

Therapist: And what things happened that made it a '4?'

Mom: Well, I *did* yell a lot and turn off his video game twice, and everything just like he said. But what Marcus *didn't* tell you is that the reason I did those things is because he didn't do a single thing he promised in session last week.

Therapist: Okay, so I guess the week didn't move from a '4' to a '5' this week like we had hoped for, huh? Let's roll it back a notch and talk about what we can get you both to agree to that will bring that '4' to a '4.5' next time we meet. Should be a bit easier to get a '4.5' than a '5,' right? So let's go back to the stuff that needs to go differently and talk that out, okay?

If Marcos or his Mom had rated the week higher than the '4' that it was the previous week, the therapist could have highlighted what things made that '4' a little better, and how they could do those same things the following week to maybe bring the number up even higher.

Since numbers are the central measure in scaling questions, there are many ways to use this in an even simpler way for younger clients. I have used a cheap, plastic ruler with children and had them make a little dry erase marker line on the number that they rated the week so that we could wipe it off and draw a new one each time there is a change. Therapists can print out a sheet of ten check boxes or ten thumbs-up symbols and have the child color in how many (being sure to clarify what a small amount or large amount means) they think signifies how the week went. An alternate idea is to keep a small box of magnetic numbers and have the child and/or family members select one and attach it to something metal in the room.

Compliments

Compliments are a big part of the SFT therapist's "tool box." When working with kid clients, therapists should be liberal in their use of compliments. Therapists can teach parents and caregivers to find compliments that are fit for them and practice using them more regularly. The compliments are specifically targeted at sending the message that clients *do* have within their power, the ability to change. The following are some good compliments to use with clients. Let's use Marcus from above, and his empty promises of doing things that Mom asks him.

- Wow, how did you do *all* your chores this week? There were a lot of them and you had gotten pretty far behind but you were able to do them!
- I'm really impressed with how well you were able to explain what specific things made this week a '4' for you. And I'm even more impressed that this week you were able to get the rating to a "4.5."
- It sounds like you're a pretty passionate and skilled video game player.
- It sounds like Mom really found it helpful that you told her more specifically when you were able to do things."

With younger children, a simple high-five, a big smile, a thumbs up, or a "great job with that!" can work well. Please note that the compliments are not meant for flattery or for everything, just used as a tool to encourage and positively highlight efforts that the client might not be aware of.

Difference

In SFT, therapists focus a great deal on "difference." In early SFT creation, the designers found that when they asked clients about their problems (e.g.,

"I have no motivation, I'm tired and depressed and sad all of the time."), and then about what the solutions would look like (e.g., "I'd be doing social things more, smile and laugh more, feel motivation and energy."), they were very disconnected. It seemed that the problems and solutions looked so different that they were barely even related to one another. So the concept of "difference" intends to look for what is inconsistent with the problem mode. SFT therapists will often ask questions like, "So you still feel depressed this week but on Friday you said you felt a teeny bit better—what was different on Friday that made it a teeny bit better?"

The difference can come in the smallest increments and it truly doesn't matter *how* small; it's still *difference,* and difference is a step away from the problem. There are lots of ways to introduce the concept of difference to younger clients. One way is simply by explaining it as I have above. For very young clients, I like to explain it the following way:

I draw what looks like an empty garden bed on a piece of paper. Then I draw a couple of flowers in the empty lot of soil. Then I explain that I'm going to grow a beautiful wildflower garden for the hummingbirds and bees and butterflies to enjoy. Then I draw ugly brown weeds all around the two beautiful flowers until they are almost covered up and we can't see the colorful petals anymore. Then I start to add more brown weeds all over the garden bed. I pause and look very sad at the child and say, "That's going to be a *lot* of pulling up weeds in this garden if I want any of the flowers to grow there." Then I say, "*Unless*...maybe if I work on planting 100 different flowers in there by spreading a bunch of wildflower seeds all over the bed, the flowers will grow so full that *they* will end up taking over and choking out the weeds instead of the other way around!"

Drawing a bunch of colorful flowers in between all the brown weeds on the paper, I explain that sometimes we might not even need to pluck out the bad stuff if we can just plant a bunch of little good stuff so that the good overgrows the bad.

Using the garden analogy as a backdrop, the therapist can then make the goal of making lots of little "differences" (flowers) from the overgrown bad stuff (the weeds). The following vignette shows how one therapist used the garden drawing as a jumping off point with her five-year-old client, Mia:

Therapist: Okay, so here's the beautiful garden we are going to try to grow. So let's talk about what one of the "bad" things, or the "weeds" that are in your life right now.

Mia: I always get in trouble for hitting my little brother.

Therapist: Okay, so hitting your brother is the yucky weed? (*Mia nods.*) So we want to get rid of that weed, right? (*Mia nods again.*) And you've had a really hard time getting rid of that weed, haven't you?

Mia: Yes, I try and try but he makes me so mad that I want to hit him to stop him from annoying me and taking my stuff.

Therapist: Okay, Mia—what do you think about us trying to do something different this week? Instead of trying to pluck that weed of hitting and get rid of it, let's try to add different things to the situation this week and see if we can grow more flowers instead.

Mia: Okay. I can *try*. But he always bugs me and touches my stuff.

Therapist: So normally, what would you do when your brother touches your stuff?

Mia: Yell at him to go away.

Therapist: And does he go away?

Mia: No.

Therapist: So then what do you do?

Mia: Hit him to make him go away.

Therapist: And then what happens?

Mia: He goes crying to Mom and tells her I hit him and I get in trouble.

Therapist: So what could you do a teeny bit *differently* when he's bugging you and touching your stuff?

Mia: Like what?

Therapist: Well maybe you could warn him? Like say, "I asked you not to touch my stuff and I don't want to get angry and hit you so can you *please* go away and play with your own stuff?"

Mia: Yeah, I could say that.

Therapist: So that would be *different* from how you usually act, right? Maybe that's like planting a flower? What's another flower you could plant?

Mia: Maybe give him my banana-shaped popper. He loves to play with that one and I have a better one now anyway.

Therapist: Yup! Sounds like another flower to me! How about this week we see what happens if we don't think about the hitting but focus on how many flowers you can plant this week with your brother and maybe those flowers will overgrow the weed.

In the next session, the therapist begins the session by asking, "So what were you able to do differently this week?" At the end of the session exploring some of the "flowers" Mia had successfully "planted," the therapist peeled off a little flower sticker and put it on the tip of Mia's nose and gave her a compliment— "You were a really great flower planter this week, Mia!"

Clients Are Experts on Their Own Lives

SFT therapists believe that clients are the experts on their own lives, so they are careful to not be directive, but rather, regularly invite clients to check in for their thoughts and the accuracy of the therapists' thoughts. When working with young clients, it's important to check in with them on if you are on the same page and if you are "getting" them.

One of the easiest ways to set a foundation for clients' expertise is to always "ask" instead of "tell" your clients things. For example, instead of saying, "So you should only use kind words when you talk to your brother this week," the therapist might ask, "So do you think that maybe it's a good idea to try using some kinder words with your brother this week and see if anything changes?" This elicits both collaboration with the client (and "buy in" is important for therapeutic success) and letting the client put the final stamp of approval on the idea (more likely that the client will do it if they agree with it).

Other ideas for phrases to use for the SFT therapist wanting to value and highlight the client's expertise on themselves are

- "Tell me if I'm way off base here, but I'm thinking that..."
- "I wonder if you think it's a good idea to..."
- "I have an idea that might be helpful here—let me know if you're on board with trying to do it this way..."
- "What do you think might be a good idea for how to talk differently to your brother?"

Do-Able Goals

Like all therapists, SFT therapists want to set up their clients for success, not failure. One way to do this is by setting very small, tangible, do-able tasks and goals in treatment that are *likely* to be able to be achieved by the client. If goals are too big, the client may fail to be able to do them, thus creating the potential failure cycle that includes dangerous ideas for impressionable young clients. These thoughts might include defeatist themes like, "It's too hard," or, "I can't do it," or, "I'll never be better." Small, tangible goals increase the chances of success for the client achieving them. And remember, in SFT, the tiniest change or "difference" is a step in the right, solution-focused direction!

Examples of small, tangible, do-able goals might include, "How about if we aim for *one* time this week, using just *one* nice word to your brother?" or, "How about we try to have you not focus on *doing* anything different this week, but just *thinking* about a nicer way to say something to your brother?" Of course, if the child comes in having surpassed the small goal and had stellar performance during the week, no one will be disappointed. Ann SFT compliment of "Wow! Great job—how were you able to figure out how to say *so* many nice things this week?" is all that is needed here.

"Formula First Session Task"

The formula first session task is a lot more simple than it sounds. This technique builds upon the SFT assumption that there are good things, progress, or exceptions happening at home, outside of the session. The easiest way to incorporate this task into therapy is as a "homework" assignment you send the child/family home with at the end of the session.

A note on "homework"— "Homework" is common in most models of therapy, as it "boils down" the entirety of the session into a basic theme or task that the clients will take away from the session and focus on in the following week between sessions. Many times, especially with young clients who may have immature memory or information organization skills, clients will spend the week after a session not remembering or even thinking at all about what was talked about or what they might be thinking or doing differently.

Remember that the term "homework" may come with a negative connotation for many kids who aren't a fan of the kind sent home from school. For this reason, it is especially important for therapists to make the homework *fun*. Some ideas are as follows:

- Stapling together a few pieces of colorful, printed cardstock paper and sending the child home with a sparkly pen to journal on the pages with.
- Including some active and fun parts of the homework like running around of the outside of the house three times when feeling frustrated.
- Sending children home with simple, drawn-out instructions for the homework. For example, the therapist can write, 1. Breathe (with a drawing of a face with puffed-out cheeks and curly cues of air coming out of the pursed lips), and 2. Think of ice cream (drawing a colorful cone with a scoop of the child's favorite flavor on top.)
- Practicing a positive phrase like, "I can do this—I'm stronger than I think I am," several times in session and then having adults in the household help the child repeat it every day. I once had a pre-teen write, "Not every day is a bad one," in the steamed-up mirror in her bathroom when she got out of the shower each morning. This exception-based homework assignment ended up being not only her favorite one, but also the most helpful one in increasing her positive outlook, confidence, and successful efforts socially at school.

A typical homework assignment for a young client (like Treyvon with the "up in your face" classmate problem) using the formula first session task would be some variation of this: "So this week, let's look around you and notice when you see that kid minding his own business," or, "Focus this week on the things other than that kid that *don't* annoy you at school," or, "When you're at school this week, notice the times when you are able to not be bother by Mr. All-up-in-your-face."

For younger clients, therapists can create a simple document to print off for the client to take home to track whatever it is the therapist wants them to look for. It can include topic areas, days of the week, lists of behaviors, or check-off boxes. Making a blank one with lines to fill in specifics for the unique homework created for each different client will save time and energy.

Case Example

Ashley was a five-year-old girl in foster care for the last two years with a retired grandma named Sally. Sally reports not having had any real issues with Ashley until she entered Kindergarten this year. Sally reports that she has been getting teacher calls that Ashley has been refusing to follow directions or participate in any academic activities at school.

A Solution-Focused Therapist's Intervention by "Mariana"

Therapist: Ashley, tell me about what happened at the reading circle this week.

Ashley: I didn't go.

Therapist: Do you like reading circles?

Ashley: Sometimes.

Therapist: Can you tell me about the times when you *do* like reading circles? What's different on those days?

Ashley: I like it when Kaia isn't next to me.

Therapist: Ahhhhh! So if you were to rate reading circle days when Kaia isn't sitting next to you, can you pick a colored marker and circle the number on the whiteboard? You can choose 1–2–3–4–5–6–7–8–9- or 10. (*The therapist writes out all of the numbers on the board and explains what they mean. Ashley circles the 9.*) Okay, and now can you circle the number of how the days are when Kaia *does* sit next to you? (*Ashley circles the 2.*)

Therapist: Hmmm…what's different on the days when Kaia sits next to you and when she doesn't?

Ashley: Kaia gets me in trouble.

Therapist: How does Kaia get you in trouble?

Ashley: Kaia makes noises and blames it on me, she takes all the turns, and bumps into me purposely. And then I get in trouble.

Therapist: Why do you get in trouble?

Ashley: Because I usually push her back or yell, "STOP!"

Therapist: Have you talked to your teacher about this?

Ashley: No.

Therapist: Why not?

Ashley: She wouldn't believe me.

Therapist: Why do you think she wouldn't believe you?

Ashley: Because I lied to her about something else another time and now she thinks I'm a liar.

Therapist: Hmmm…this is a *lot* of problem talk, Ashley—getting in trouble, thinking the teacher sees you as a liar, not liking reading circle, getting pushed up against by Kaia. That must feel pretty bad, huh? (*Ashley nods.*)

Therapist: So I want for us to see if we can come up with some fixes for some of these problems. Will you help me? (*Ashley nods.*) Can you come sit next to me and help me write down some ideas for what we might be able to try differently this week?

The following week, the therapist had Ashley circle the number of the week in a different color and reading circle had moved from a '2' when Kaia sat next to her, to a '4.' Ashley had tried asking Kaia nicely to not push up against her leg and Kaia had said, "Sorry" and stopped. Ashley (with the help of Sally) had gone to school early one morning to talk to the teacher. Sally had also arranged a fun playdate for Ashley and Kaia to go mini-golfing and out for ice cream the following weekend which Ashley was really excited for.

Key Takeaways

Solution-Focused Therapy (SFT) will always center on a few key concepts when using the model in playful interventions. The following are a few key elements to remember when working from an SFT-informed lens:

- This model is known for its focus on *solution building,* instead of on *problem saturation* in therapy. For SFT-influenced therapists, solution building can be infused into sessions by the choice of language, focusing on exceptions (times when the problem is *not* present), and playful interventions. The SFT-based therapist should be sure to include the focus on the present and future instead of on the past during discussions in sessions whenever possible.
- SFT therapists believe that clients only need a *small* change in order for the "snowball effect" to organically create bigger changes.
- Playful activities that center on the notions of The Miracle Question, scaling, and exceptions can be especially fun and meaningful for younger clients and help them understand the power of these concepts in building solutions.

8   Cognitive Behavioral Therapy (CBT)

Model Background and Key Concepts

Dr. Aaron Beck is the most notable figure associated with the creation of the Cognitive Behavioral Therapy (CBT) model. CBT solidified as a "model" in the 1960s and 1970s (e.g., Beck, et al., 1979; Friedberg 2006), but it has evolved over time and adapted to include new research and more modern views on treatment. Although not generally seen as a "systemic" model like the others provided in the text thus far, my reasons for including it are twofold. First, CBT is practiced in most agencies and mental health facilities and is generally accepted as being a solid, evidence-based model. Since it is so common, most therapists will encounter or be trained in CBT at some point in their careers. Second, CBT lends itself so well to playful interventions with young clients.

The model aims to help clients recognize how problematic or faulty thinking can influence their actions. CBT posits that problems are caused by four main things—faulty patterns of thinking, learned and ingrained patterns of thinking (that have become "habit"), inaccurate perceptions of self and others, and the lack of adequate coping tools to deal with the above. CBT therapists look to heighten awareness of these areas for clients and to highlight the ways in which they contribute to problematic areas. Additionally, therapists will work with clients to build better "toolboxes" of strategies to use in working through these areas.

Please note that with this model, there are countless resources for CBT activities with younger clients; the ones I offer here are the "tip of the iceberg" and only reflect some of the ones I have creatively used in my practice that have been particularly helpful. If the ones I offer below resonate with you, I encourage you to read more from the many sources of everything CBT. You can find things I haven't covered here (like responsibility pie charts and various worksheets) online.

Playful Technique Ideas

Explaining "CBT"

Therapists can begin sessions with kid clients and/or their families by explaining what CBT is in the simplest terms. Start by choosing one member of the family

DOI: 10.4324/9781003506072-9

(e.g., Mom) and asking the child client, "So if your Mom were to jump up suddenly and run out of the room right now, what might be some of the reasons why she would do that?" Read the following vignette of how the therapist explains CBT via the lens of this question:

Client: She has to go to the bathroom?
Therapist: Yes! Maybe she drank a LOT of water on her way here. What else?
Client: She has to throw up?
Therapist: Another good one! What else?
Client: I can't think of any more.
Therapist: Okay, what about if she had to make an emergency phone call? What if she felt really upset about something? What if something I said really offended her?
Client: What if she had *ants* in her *pants?*
Therapist: Yes! Ants in her pants would *not* be good, huh? So you see, when a person *does* something, like jumping up suddenly and leaving the room, there is a reason inside their head that tells them they should do that action. So for mom, maybe her thoughts are telling her, "I feel really sick and I might throw up and I don't want to do it in the therapy office so I better jump up and run to the bathroom."
Client: Yeah, that's a smart thing to think.
Therapist: But sometimes it works the *other* way too. So, what if Mom was sitting there, looking uncomfortable with a frown on her face but *didn't* jump up suddenly and run out of the room? Maybe her *staying* in the room was because her thoughts told her *not* to act, *not* to jump up and run because it would be rude to leave so suddenly, or maybe she thought she had a bit more time before she actually threw up and was trying to finish the session to be nice?
Client: (*Laughs.*)
Therapist: So see what I'm getting at here? What we *think* often is behind we choose certain actions. And how we *act* often makes us have thoughts about it. They go hand-in-hand and are always telling each other what to do or think.

This explanation can be the foundation of everything else that is talked about or built upon in therapy. Asking the client and/or family about what they were thinking that "told" them to do certain things, and what they were thinking about the action they took should be regularly interspersed in CBT treatment.

Generalization

In CBT, the process of "generalization" can often get in the way of how clients think and act. For example, if 10-year-old client "Holly" tells you that her brother *never* lets her play video games with him and gets mad *all the time* when she asks him, she might be generalizing a few encounters to the "fact" that he won't let her. She thereby is relegated to feeling disappointed and sad and ultimately, will stop asking him to play. Likewise, if Holly has tried to play with a few kids at school and she perceived them as rejecting her, she might generalize this experience to the thought that, "No one likes me. No one wants to play with me."

One playful way to help kid clients understand generalization is by stressing words like *always* and *never* during their treatment. For example, read the following vignette to see how the therapist uses the emphasis of generalizing words to challenge Holly's faulty perceptions:

Therapist: So tell me how it went this week when you tried our new strategy for trying to play with the kids in the neighborhood.

Holly: Well, they were all playing outside at the end of the road with bikes and sidewalk chalk and they were making like, obstacle courses to run through and rides bikes around. But no one asked me to play with them.

Therapist: Okay, did that seem fun to you? Like something you'd want to join in on?

Holly: Yes! It was better than sitting in the house with no screens—I'm not allowed to have my tablet until after dinner.

Therapist: Okay, so how did you approach them?

Holly: I just walked up and stood there.

Therapist: And then what?

Holly: No one talked to me.

Therapist: Did you say anything to any of the kids?

Holly: No.

Therapist: So *no one* said a word to you? At *all*?

Holly: Well one girl said, "Hi." But that's it.

Therapist: So it's not really *no one* who said anything to you, but *one* person did, and *most* of them didn't, right?

Holly: Yeah, I guess so.

Therapist: So what did you do then?

Holly: I did what you said to do. I tried to help by picking up some of the balls and throwing them back to them when they missed catching them. And I put the orange cones back upright when they knocked them over with the bikes.

Therapist: And then what?

Holly: A few of them said, "Thanks." But no one asked me to play.

Therapist: Okay, wait a minute here! So *no one* asked you to play, but *some* of them said things to you, and *some* of them did not? (*Holly nods.*) And *then* what happened?

Holly: I just kept doing that for a while and then one girl said I could use her bike while she was playing tag. But I didn't have a helmet so I didn't. But I sat on a skateboard and just scooted around for a while.

Therapist: Hmmmmm, so Holly, do you think that maybe the key here is that no one has to *ask* you to play but that you just kind of start doing it?

The therapist here was able to reframe the situation for Holly, but also ease into the discussion by highlighting the generalizations she was making. This allowed openings for possibilities in her thinking, and thereby potential new actions.

Another great way to use the common generalizing words (e.g., always, never, one, all) is to write each one on an index card and laminate them. I like to add a few extra cards with better qualifying words on them as well (e.g., everyone, some, a few, most, sometimes, often). The therapist can use the cards to help child clients make choices about which words/descriptors actually are the most fitting for the situation.

Reinforcement

Reinforcement is something that increases the probability that a desired response or a specific behavior will happen again in the future. The use of reinforcement is a powerful tool for CBT therapists to use. The inclusion of parent(s) or guardian(s) in sessions is a great way to model how reinforcement can be used to help kid clients.

The simplest and most fun ways to reinforce are by using rewards for positive movements by the child or family. The key is in discovering which rewards or reinforcers will work best for each individual client. For example, some kids respond really well to simply hearing compliments, praise, or encouraging, positive feedback. In this case, "Great job!" or, "You managed that situation really well!" are enough. For other kids, hugs or high-fives from parents or guardians are possibilities. Token "gifts," especially ones that contribute to or enhance the therapy, are great choices. For example, I have purchased inexpensive, colorful, bulk mini-notebooks online, affirmation cards, little figurines, and stickers, and painted rocks with inspirational words or reminders on them over the years. Individually wrapped candy can work as well, but it is important to ask parents/guardians before introducing these foods/sweets as a motivator is okay with them.

By far, the best reinforcer that I have ever used with kid clients and/or their families is what I call the "reward jar." It is simply any empty bowl, jar, or other container that a family has around the house. The therapist helps the child client (after checking with the parent or guardian first) create a list of things they really enjoy and would see as rewards to work toward. The therapist writes down each thing on a tiny piece of paper, folds it up into a tiny square, and puts them all in the jar. Once a client has reached the desired behavior, the child can choose one of the pieces of paper as a reward and reinforcer.

This activity can be done at home (with things like staying up an hour later, going out for ice cream, taking the dog to the dog park, having a friend over, getting to choose what's for dinner one night, an extra half hour of screen time) or in the therapist's office (with things like going for a jog around the building together first, choosing the game or activity to play, making up a silly dance the therapist has to do, choosing and writing the week's inspirational quote on the therapist's whiteboard with colored dry erase markers). The younger the client, the more effective the simplest things are.

Reinforcers can also be things a child client takes home to remind them to stay on track. Stickers, affirmation cards, or simply writing a surprise little note to the client to take home and read *only* when they feel they aren't doing well or have fallen off track. Putting a sticky note on the bathroom mirror at home with a positive note of reinforcement can be a helpful reminder and motivator when the client looks at it at least twice every day.

Behavior Assignments

Behavior assignments are similar to the concept of "homework" that therapists practicing many different models use. They use this to help the child continue the important parts of therapy outside of the session and to integrate those activities and themes into their real lives at home and at school.

Behavior assignments or homework can be just about anything the therapist thinks would be helpful for the child client and/or family members to practice at home. One way for the therapist to do this is to assign each family member a task for the week. It can be anything from "Putting your dishes in the dishwasher without being asked," to "Practice taking deep breaths before you respond to a question that is annoying to you." It is a really good idea to write down each task on a sticky note to send home with the client/family, as it is easy to forget what the homework was during the busy week. Make sure to check in with clients on if they are willing to do the homework and if they think the homework is fitting and might be helpful. This checking-in will both serve as making the assignment collaborative, as well as increasing the likelihood of the child/family doing it if you have their buy-in to the idea.

Playful ways to assign homework when doing family work is to ask family members to assign themselves a behavioral assignment for the week. If someone gets "stuck" and can't come up with anything, the other family members can come up with ideas to help them out. The therapist can also help out by helping generate suggestions. If there is a family member who doesn't really need to work on anything, or the family has just come through some intense times and needs a break, the therapist can give playful assignments like, "Laugh more," or, "Wear something purple this week."

The "3 C's"

The 3 C's is a favorite activity to use with young clients. CBT has many different strategies like this one, but I have found this one to be the simplest and most helpful in my work with young clients and/or their families.

- "Catch it" This is helping clients be more aware of the unconscious negative thoughts that can show up out of habit. One example might be, "Everybody thinks I'm ugly." The first step in reframing or coping better with negative thoughts is to "catch" the thoughts when they first occur.
- "Check it" The therapist can help clients to check the reality of their negative thoughts by asking some clarifying questions about the thoughts. For example, "Do you think it's accurate that *everybody* thinks you're ugly? How does it help you to walk around thinking that everyone thinks you're ugly?"
- "Change it" The therapist can help clients to create slight variations of their negative thoughts by restating them in a less distorted way. For example,

I heard some girls at school say I was ugly. There could be a lot of reasons they would say that—to hurt me, make fun of me, make me feel bad, or because they're jealous or angry about my choice to dress differently. I know that some people *don't* think I'm ugly. My best friend always tells me I have the sweetest smile and striking eyes, and my sister says she wishes she looked more like me.

The vignette at the end of the chapter will demonstrate further how the 3 C's can be a therapy staple in treatment with kid clients.

Journaling

Journaling is a cornerstone of CBT activities and there are many ways to utilize this activity. To make it more fun, therapists can order inexpensive, whimsical bulk journals online to give to kid clients, or for a cheaper alternative, just staple a bunch of sheets of paper together and let the child label the front with their name and, "My Journal," and decorate it with coloring or stickers. The journal can either be kept at home, in the therapist's office for use in session or can be brought back and forth. Alternatively, if parents or guardians can afford it and are willing, they can take the child to the store to buy a blank journal of their choosing.

The following are some ways to use the journal:

- To record feelings or actions during the week. A popular use here is for the client to write down "bad" or negative thoughts and then write a more positive one next to it. For example, a child might write, "Angry that Dad wouldn't let me buy a new video game," and could write after it, "I don't always get what I want when I want it, but my birthday is coming up and I might get it then."

- The therapist can provide prompts for each week. For example, "Write a list of the things you like most about yourself."
- Writing down things that happened that the child wants to remember to talk to the therapist about.
- Writing notes to parents or guardians in the journal and giving it to them to write their responses to the child in as a way to continue and improve a healthy "dialogue" between them.
- Using the journal as a space to just draw or write or color when feeling bored or anxious or sad.
- Using the journal to record angry words and scribbles instead of acting on the emotion in a less appropriate way.
- The therapist can write down important features or themes from what was talked about the session in the journal and send it home with the client to look at or read when they need better coping strategies during the week. For example, "Remember that no matter how bad a day it was, you always get a new start tomorrow to have it be different."

It is important for therapists to ensure that family members will agree to respect the child's privacy in not looking at their journal. If the therapist or child is in doubt, the therapist can keep the journal locked away in the therapy office for use in sessions only.

"Self-Talk"

Many young clients will have negative "self-talk" that chatters away in their heads as they go through their days. Therapists can help clients identify these "voices" and give them names and colors or entities. They can begin to develop these voices and challenge them to increase the clients' awareness of both when they are chattering, and when their messages are distorted, faulty, or not helpful.

For young clients, therapists can purchase either blank colored dot stickers (the kind that might have prices on them and stuck on items at a yard sale), or just create their own faces by cutting circles out of paper, coloring them, and putting faces or names on them. For a symbolic message of these voices, I like to let the child leave the first session with a yellow, smiley face sticker stuck on one shoulder and a blue sad or angry-faced sticker on their other shoulder. I ask the child and the parents/guardians (if they are involved in treatment) to watch during the week to see how many times they all think the yellow smiley face is chatting or the blue angry face is chatting.

Externalizing the self-talk into two different voices that are separate from the child can help them to better identify when the chatter is occurring, and better understand when the voices are being helpful or not.

Exposure Therapy

This section includes just a very brief overview of how to use exposure in sessions with younger clients. There are far more expansive trainings on how to do full exposure therapy that may be a good idea if you find this simple inclusion in treatment helpful.

The idea of exposure is that when a child has a specific fear or generalized anxiety about something, the therapy room can be a safe space to be exposed to teeny, tiny bits of scary things without being upset or feeling overwhelmed. I also like using exposure because it demonstrates to the child that they have some control and ability to face the fear without getting too upset.

Let's say that four-year-old Li is afraid of dogs because her friend's dogs jumped on her and knocked her down and licked her and one accidently scratched her arm last year. The therapist can start by writing down the word "dog" in big bubble letters and let Li color them in and talk about what she is thinking and feeling when she sees the word or thinks about dogs. The therapist can act like a dog and get on the floor, pad over to Li, and put a paw up and bark. The therapist can ask Li what she thinks the dog wants—to be stroked or patted on the head? To go out? To eat? Then the therapist can talk about dogs in a different way, working with Li to list all the different kinds and colors of dogs and what their reputations or common uses are. For example, Dalmatians are black and white spotted and used to be used as guard dogs in firehouses. Next, the therapist can introduce pictures of these dogs into session so the client can look at them while still discussing their common personalities or uses. For online sessions, the therapist can share screens and can look up all sorts of shapes, sizes, and colors of dogs.

Therapists can read children's books with friendly dog characters in them during sessions or have hypothetical conversations about what it would like to have a dog as a pet—getting up early to let it go out, walking it in the rain, what to feed it, if it would be allowed on furniture or the bed, what some good dog names would be. Therapists can also help the child clients with visualizations and imagery activities about dogs, but reminding the child they can exit the thought games whenever they feel anxious.

When the therapist feels like Li is ready, the parents or guardians might take her to a pond where Li can see dogs and watch them bark and play, but behind cages and fences. It's important that therapists check in with clients on how they are feeling while doing each step of the exposure, and they can dial it back to the previous stage if the child seems too anxious.

Relaxation

More recently, some CBT therapists have integrated other modalities into their work to maximize the clients' ability to recognize certain things like intrusive or distorted thoughts and patterns of thinking and perception. Relaxation, meditation, imagery, and mindfulness are all quite conducive to working with child clients. They can easily be made playful and fun, and they also offer strategies that the children can use throughout their lives. For this section, I will focus on relaxation. You can find more ideas on the other items listed above in the "General Interventions" chapter of the text.

Therapists can begin and end each session with a very short relaxation exercise to help child clients form the habit of knowing how to calm themselves and be able to better focus on their thoughts and feelings. Have the client lie down and close their eyes if they are comfortable doing so. Focus first on their breathing,

Some children may be too young or have attention issues that make it difficult for them to be still for this activity. In these cases, the therapist can offer some faster-paced imagery or give the child some small movement task to do while focusing on the activity. The following are a few examples a therapist uses with five-year-old Jezebel:

- "Okay Jezebel, I see your eyes opening a lot, so let's try this—I want you to open and close your eyes while you are listening to my voice, but I want you to try to open and close them to match your breathing. So when you breathe in (therapist inhales dramatically) your eyes should be open, and then close them while you breathe out (therapist exhales slowly)."
- "Now while your eyes are closed Jezebel, I want you to imagine each of the words that I say in your mind, okay? (Therapist begins listing words quickly and then goes more slowly after several words/phrases.) *Elephant. Gray. Loud. Playing. Other animals. Playing together. Mama elephant. Angry."* In this scenario, the therapist has the ability to layer words that may be more activating to the child with words or phrases that will likely evoke more calming visualizations.
- "We are going to play the 1-to-10 game like we do at the beginning and end of every session, okay? So as a reminder, you lie down and get comfy and I'm going to count down from 10 and you have to do is relax your body and listen to my voice. *10—Your body feels full of cloudy, smoky anger. 9—Breathe in deeply and then let it out, letting a little swirl of anger smoke leave your body. 8—As you take another breath in, imagine the bright yellow sunlight coming into your body, relaxing you."* And so on.

Case Example

Rae is a 12-year-old non-binary pre-teen who presents with anxiety and school refusal. Their parents are recently divorced and Rae refuses to see their mother, as she will not call her daughter by their chosen name of "Rae," but rather calls them by their birth name, "Helena."

A Cognitive Behavioral Therapist's Intervention by "Kim"

The therapist had met with the entire family (mom, dad, and Rae) the previous year when the parents were going through a divorce. Since Rae began having problems with going to school and increased anxiety, they refused to have the parents attend sessions with them. The therapist continued to try to encourage Rae to have at least their mother attend one session so the therapist could help work on their relationship, but they refused. The following is a snippet from one of Kim's individual sessions with Rae:

Therapist: So Rae, tell me about how the week has been.

Rae: I went to school on Monday and Tuesday, but I just couldn't do the rest of the week. My mother kept texting me on Tuesday night and I just couldn't go the next morning.

Therapist: What did your mom have to say?

Rae: More of the same old crap. About how I was born a girl and that there's no such thing as non-binary. And that I was named after my great grandmother and that it was so disrespectful of her to not keep my given name.

Therapist: Hmmmm…so how did you respond to her?

Rae: I didn't.

Therapist: So then did she stop texting eventually?

Rae: Yes. She gave up after like, an hour. She freaking *hates* me. I bet she wishes I was never even born. I'm such a disgrace to her. Yet I'm supposed to wanna *see* her?

Therapist: Well, can we start with our favorite 3 C's activity for a second? (*Rae nods.*) So your mom *hates* you, wishes you were never born, and thinks you're a disgrace?

Rae: Pretty much.

Therapist: Okay, I'm going to ask you to "catch" that thought for a minute. Got it? (*Rae nods.*) Okay, now let's check it. Could there be another explanation here?

Rae: Probably not. Pretty sure she hates me.

Therapist: Can I help you out here? You let me know if any of these seem like possibilities, okay? Maybe your mom just doesn't understand any of this? Maybe she's frustrated with not having things be different? Maybe she has her own guilt about needing to maintain an allegiance to your great grandmother by keeping that name, and it has nothing to do with you?

Rae: Well, yeah, some of that's probably right. Like she definitely doesn't understand me. And she is all "old school" with names and values and stuff. And she is kind of a control freak.

Therapist: Okay, so maybe we can change the negative thought we caught to something a bit different? Can you think of something?

Rae: Okay, maybe she doesn't hate *me* but does hate that I want to be different from her.

Therapist: Yeah, I think that's probably more accurate. I guess if she really hated you, she wouldn't keep trying to see you or text you, huh?

Rae: I guess.

Therapist: So I have some homework for you this week if you're game? (*Rae nods.*) How about if you jot down a couple of negative thoughts you have this week in your journal—you know, ones like, "My mother hates me." And after each one, try to think about how true the thought is and how/if it's helpful to you, and then write a "change it" statement after each one that is maybe a bit more valid.

Rae: Okay. I love journaling anyway. And that's a good idea I guess. I know I beat up on myself a lot with how I think. Can I draw on those pages too?

Therapist: Absolutely! Sometimes drawings and doodles speak far louder than words. I'd love to see your artwork if you feel like showing it to me next week.

Key Takeaways

Cognitive Behavioral Therapy (CBT) will always center on a few key concepts when using the model in playful interventions. The following are a few key elements to remember when working from a CBT-informed lens:

- The CBT model aims to help clients recognize how problematic or faulty thinking can influence their actions. Therapists can work playfully with clients to build better "toolboxes" of strategies to use in working through areas of how thinking informs behavior.
- Therapists who work Cognitive Behaviorally might find it helpful to focus on how clients can (faultily) generalize thoughts and events to other situations, and how reinforcement influences why/how clients might do things.
- CBT-influenced therapists have many helpful tools to use with younger clients. These include things like playful "homework assignments, journaling, and listening to "self-talk."

9 Integrative Systemic Therapy (IST)

Framework Background and Key Concepts

Unlike the *models* I've presented in the previous chapters, IST is a *framework* (Russell et al., 2023; Pinsof et al., 2018) from which therapists can draw when navigating the course of therapy with a client. Many of the central themes and concepts lend themselves well to work with younger clients. Since IST is a framework, those using it adhere to the notion that no one model of treatment is best. Rather, the framework allows for any number of strategies and interventions to be chosen based on the therapist's and client's assessment of the problem sequences and the areas that contribute to constraints.

IST centers on the idea that there are three main parts to therapy—locating a problem in a problem sequence, finding possible solution sequences, and the possibility of constraints standing in the way of successful outcomes in treatment. IST adheres to a systemic view that shuns linear causality in favor of a more recursive view of how problems arise, and a preference for doing work within the context of family whenever possible. Thus, problems always occur within a problem *sequence*. Once the problem sequence is discovered and understood, the therapist can help clients move toward possible solution sequences. If the transition from problem to solution fails to go swimmingly, the therapist will then look for the possible *constraints* that serve as "roadblocks" to alleviating the problem. These constraints can also include factors related to things like culture or family organization. The framework provides therapists with a decision-making structure that suggests when they should borrow from other models of therapy.

The following will offer some creative and playful ways to integrate some of the language and tenets of the IST framework that can help young clients and their families work toward change. If the following concepts resonate with you, I urge you to seek out one of the great texts or training on IST for much more information on framing therapy, families, and change.

DOI: 10.4324/9781003506072-10

Playful Technique Ideas

Alliance Priority Guideline

As with most types of modern treatment, the therapist-client relationship is paramount. IST has a number of "guidelines," one of which is the "Alliance Priority Guideline." Understanding the importance of monitoring and maintaining a strong therapeutic alliance is key to doing any effective therapy. During treatment, therapists should be checking in on the "health" of the relationship on a regular basis.

There are many playful ways to do "check ins" with younger clients. Using the thumbs up/thumbs down action for assessing the client's buy-in is great, and the icon for this motion is included on many teletherapy platforms as well. Another helpful phrase is simply asking clients, "What do you think? Are we in agreement? Are we on the same page?"

If therapists are ever unsure of or concerned about movement or progress in therapy, this guideline suggests that attending to the strength of the relationship is a vital area to assess.

Non-summativity/Perspectivism

IST borrows a great deal from early systemic work and views, the bedrock of the field of Marriage and Family Therapy. One such concept is called "non-summativity" that IST uses to build the idea of "perspectivism." This can be particularly helpful to young clients in understanding that we never have the "whole story" on things. A fun way to introduce this concept to younger clients is to share with them the "math" problem of $1 + 1 = 3$. Of course, at first they laugh and (accurately) tell the therapist that the equation is completely wrong. *Everybody* knows that $1 + 1 = 2$! We all have our own unique views and understanding of things, and those are limited.

For example, consider the following vignette between the therapist and a 12-year-old client Grayson. Grayson has Autism Spectrum Disorder (ASD) and presents with a difficult time with social interactions and tolerance of other children's behaviors. The therapist attempts to use the concept of non-summativity to help Grayson see the "background" that may exist outside of the limited picture he paints:

Therapist: Tell me what's been going on at school this week, Grayson.
Grayson: Same old stuff. Kids being annoying. Teachers being dumb.
Therapist: Why are the kids annoying?
Grayson: Because they are too loud.
Therapist: And why are the teachers dumb?
Grayson: Because they don't care. They don't do anything about the yelling and screaming and laughing too loud.
Therapist: SO you think the teachers don't care?

Grayson: They don't care that it bothers me.
Therapist: So you've talked to the teachers and let them know how the loudness feels to you?
Grayson: No.
Therapist: Hmmmmm...so I wonder how they would know it bothered you then?
Grayson: Duhhhhh! It's loud and annoying, they *have* to know that, they have ears, they can hear it.
Therapist: So remember how we talked about $1 + 1 = 3$ last week? (*Grayson nods.*) And how when we think about things, we don't always have *all* the information? So if we add up all the parts—kids loud, teachers hear the annoying sounds, teachers don't do anything about it, teachers don't care that it bothers you—it doesn't really make sense does it?
Grayson: No, it doesn't. That's why they are dumb.
Therapist: Maybe we are missing something here, Grayson? What else are we missing from the $1 + 1$ equation that could help us understand why the teachers don't care?
Grayson: Dunno.
Therapist: How about this—tell me what you think. Maybe what's missing is that even though the teachers hear the noise, it doesn't bother them. Maybe they are used to noise since they are teachers and are around a lot of kids every day. (*Grayson shrugs.*) Maybe the teachers don't know the sound bothers you because you've never told them. Maybe they think you are okay with it because you always seem content reading a book at recess when the other kids are being loud. Maybe some kids need to let out some noise since they have to be quiet in classes all day and feel like they will explode if they don't let it out.

Going along with the idea of non-summativity above, "perspectivism" describes that what we "know" about something is necessarily limited by the individual perspective from which any one person views it. Therapists can also introduce and use the word "perspective" or "point of view" on a regular basis to help younger clients understand that there is no singular "truth," but rather lots of different "truths" depending on one's viewpoint. Doing this can help kid clients resist personalizing things that happen with others, and help them try instead to look at different points of view to increase understanding.

Candy Jar Analogy

Whether with a real candy jar, a drawn and colored one, or with just the verbal description, the candy jar analogy is a super simple and powerful way to help set the stage for kid clients and their families. Think about a candy jar filled with different kinds of candies. There's no need to struggle to dig way down deep into the jar when there are plenty of candies that can easily be swiped from the top of the jar. So too are how the IST therapist views problems and solutions. Start at the top with the easiest broad brush strokes. For example, in the above example of 12-year-old Grayson, top of the candy jar was the therapist focusing on solutions to the problem that included the simplest things like, "Did you tell your teachers how the noise bothers you?" or "What are some of the things we might be missing when looking at this situation?" Potentially "easy" solutions that might quickly lead to improvement for Grayson.

Conversely, there are indeed times when we might need to work harder and dig deeper into the candy jar to find information and solutions. For example, with a real candy jar, we may want a certain kind or color of candy that resides deeper in the jar. Maybe one of the red sour ones is near the top and the chocolate ones at the bottom, so we dig deeper to get the chocolate one because that is the one we feel like today. Likewise, if the top of the candy jar attempts at finding "easy" solutions to problems are not working, it may be time to dig deeper for another kind.

Therapists can use the candy jar analogy to playfully challenge kid clients about what the "easier" fixes might be, and when there might be deeper stuff to explore. I recently asked a kid client, "So what do you think? Is this going be a top of the candy jar or bottom of the candy jar problem?" The client replied, "Oh it's a really deep, bottom of the jar problem. Wait until you hear how bad it is." By the end of the session, we were able to collectively agree that although there were some complicated dynamics of substance use history and depression for this client that couldn't really understand (deeper in the jar stuff like family history of addiction and bipolar diagnoses), there were several things that were top of the jar and he was readily able to tackle (strategies to go to bed earlier, hanging around different peers, having some family therapy sessions with his mom).

Problem Sequences

Problem sequences are one way to describe the circularity of how human interactions can lead to problematic or dysfunctional patterns. Helping child clients understand the idea of problem sequences is helpful in two really important ways. First, it externalizes the "problem" into a pattern or sequence that lives *outside* of the child, but of which the child can still have an active part. Secondly, seeing a problem as not simply a stand-alone entity, but rather as embedded *within* interactions creates a less blaming or pathologizing environment. Both of these ways help younger clients and/or their families view problems in a systemic manner, while increasing empowerment and decreasing fault.

One easy way to introduce what problem sequences are and how they work is to have a child clients choose figurines or stuffed animals or dolls in the office to represent both themselves and all the members of their family. If the issues that arise are occurring at school or socially in the neighborhood, for example, the child can choose to represent those school or social players rather than family members.

Let's take the six-year-old client, Max, who is having some playground issues with other kids. The therapist leads this activity by asking Max to talk about how a particularly good or bad day went during the week. The therapist can prompt him by maneuvering a pencil, ruler, or some other item that can be used to point at each of the selected characters as Max tells the story. If he gets stuck in a linear way (for example, "I got really mad at my friend, Joseph!"), the therapist can then point to the "Joseph" figure and ask, "And then what did Joseph do?" to help continue highlighting the sequencing.

*A note to therapists--using a tiny sticky note to label each character by name that the child chooses for friends or family members will greatly help you re-member who is who during this activity.

Solution Sequences

After uncovering the sequence in which a problem is embedded, it is fairly easy to begin generating solution sequences, or possible fixes to the problem. After therapists help younger clients and/or their families see and understand the problem sequences, it is time to help them see how solution sequences work in much the same way. Consider the following vignette between the therapist and the six-year-old client, Max (above):

Therapist: Okay Max, so you said you got really mad at your friend Joseph? (*pointing to the "Max" figurine*). So when you got mad, then what did Joseph do? (*pointing to the "Joseph" figurine*).

Max: He got mad back at me.

Therapist: And then what did *you* do, Max? (*pointing again at the "Max" figurine*).

Max: Then the teacher came over and made us go sit on opposite sides of the outside wall.

Therapist: Oops, we don't have a "teacher" figurine—could you go choose another figurine and I'll put "teacher" on a little sticky so we know which one the teacher is? (*Max chooses a little duck in red, rubber boots*).

Max: And then are you gonna ask me what I did after that?

Therapist: Yes! That's really good—you figured out my game!

Max: Then I got really sad.

Therapist: So let's try something a little different now with the figurines, okay? We just showed how the *problem* went, so now let's try to figure out how the *solution* might have worked out.

Max: What do you mean?

Therapist: Well, let's start with you, Max. (*Pointing at the "Max" figurine*).

Max: Okay.

Therapist: So what could you have done differently that maybe could have fixed the problem? (*Pointing at "Max" figurine*).

Max: Like not yelled at Joseph?
Therapist: Yup. That's a good one. And if you hadn't yelled at Joseph, then what would he have done? (*Pointing to the "Joseph" figurine*).
Max: Probably asked me to play.
Therapist: Okay. And what could Joseph have done differently that might have fixed the problem of why you were mad at him? (*Pointing to the "Joseph" figurine*).
Max: Well, if he didn't call me a "dummy" for dropping the ball then I wouldn't have gotten mad at him.
Therapist: Wow—these are lots of great solutions so far!

Constraints

Constraints exist as a rationale for why perhaps an attempted solution sequence (like Max not yelling at Joseph above) doesn't work. Another word for constraints that I like to use with younger clients is the work "roadblocks." There are many versions of mini orange traffic cones or roadblock simulation toys online that can be effective tools for therapists to help kid clients visualize the impasses that can sometimes exist between people. For an even simpler manipulative, therapists can draw a basic triangle or cone shape, cut it out, and color it bright orange. This little handmade cutout can be placed between the figurines (a.k.a., family members or friends) when the discussions of possible solutions (a.k.a., not yelling, not calling someone a "dummy") do not seem to yield improvement or change.

Therapists can pepper explorations of problem sequences and attempted solution sequences with comments like, "So what do you think the roadblock is here for you two?" or, "What's constraining you or holding you back from getting along better with Joseph?" The simple terms and language therapists can teach child clients and their families when looking at and understanding problems and solutions can be something they carry as a helpful tool throughout their lives.

Positive vs. Negative Explanations

Positive and negative explanations are different ways to think about things that can offer powerful reframes for younger clients. These concepts are especially fitting with discussions with kid clients and their families about constraints.

Positive explanations are basically "why" questions. A couple of examples might be, "So why didn't you answer your mother?" or, "Why did you lie?" These types of questions usually yield more linear information and straightforward information. They also put the responsibility on the singular client for the answer.

Conversely, negative explanations would include questions like, "What stood in the way of you apologizing to your mother?" or, "What stopped you from asking the questions you really wanted to ask?" or, "What do you think is behind not having told your mother what you were really feeling?" Using questions that pull at negative explanations shifts the onus of the issue or constraint away from the client, and more toward the constraint. These questions are also less likely to be shaming or blaming and more likely to be actionable.

Consider the following two question types and the possible responses they might elicit from 13-year-old Mary who presents with having issues with her mother:

Positive Explanation Question:	Negative Explanation Question:
Why did you lie to your mother?	What stopped you from telling your mother the truth?

Possible Response:	Possible Response:
Because I can't tell her the truth.	Fear of her reaction.

You can see that Mary's response to the Positive Explanation Question yields different information than the Negative Explanation Question. Furthermore, the direction the therapist's next questions would go in differs between the two as well. For example, after Mary responds, "I can't tell her the truth," the following is how that conversation might go:

Therapist: Why can't you tell your mother the truth, Mary?
Mary: Because she wouldn't understand.
Therapist: Why do you think she wouldn't understand?
Mary: Because we are just really different people.
Therapist: And why are you two so different?
Mary: She's really controlling and judgy.

Now consider how the therapy might go from the jumping off point of Mary's response to the Negative Explanation Question, "Fear of her reaction":

Therapist: What do you think stops you from feeling comfortable in being truthful with your mother, Mary?
Mary: She's scary when she's mad. I don't want her to be angry at me.
Therapist: And what do you think gets in your mother's way of being calm with you?
Mary: She needs things to be her way.
Therapist: What do you think is behind your mother's need to have things a certain way?
Mary: She says her mom was like that with her.
Therapist: And what do you think is behind *your* need to have her not angry with you? Is she *that* scary? (*Mary laughs*).
Mary: Kinda scary, but not *that* scary. I just feel bad when I know she's angry at me. I don't want her to hate me.

Importance of "Mind"

The "how" we think about things is such a vital part of understanding problems, ourselves, and our interactions. IST-trained therapists look at the concept of "mind" as being an important thing to consider when working within systems. "Mind" in itself can be a constraint to things getting better.

For example, in the scenario above, the client Mary shared that she felt bad when her mother was angry with her because "I don't want her to hate me." Mary's belief that if her mother is angry at her, she might then hate her is a big part of the constraint to her being able to tell the truth to her mother. If Mary were able to think differently about her mother's anger at her, she might be able to be more truthful to her, and doing that might be a solution sequence that would make Mary and her mother's interactions far less stressful and negative.

IST therapists look at three specific levels of mind and label them M1, M2, and M3. This concept is super helpful in helping younger clients and/or their families understand how the way we think, feel, and believe about things can have a huge influence on our interactions.

- M1—things that the client actively expresses, like, "I'm worried about this," or, "I don't want my mother to hate me." Therapists can appropriately punctuate these with validating statements like, "Yeah, I can see how that makes you feel bad," or, "When you talk about going back to school, I can hear the worry in your voice." Other techniques to use with clients with M1 expressions are helping clients reframe their views or beliefs, think more calmly about those things, or work with them on loosening up and making their rigid narratives more malleable. They may also be able to see the sequence of thoughts and feelings and begin to question their connections or the implications of the sequence for how they feel, think, or act.
- M2—things that have a far deeper meaning to the client, like things wired from traumatic experiences, a repeated internalization of messages, or a personality disorder or other mental health diagnosis. M2 expressions may take longer and require more effort and care and support to work through. Strategies that incorporate trauma work, coordination with medical doctors, or intensive family work may be needed here. M2 is an analysis of how parts or mechanisms of mind operate and fit together.
- M3—these are parts of clients that are so deeply wired in constraints that movement just seems impossible. M3 expressions are rooted in a less-developed self. In these cases, therapists may need to slow down therapy and spend time working on foundational elements of self and realities in order to get to the point of being able to do more relational work with significant improvements in functioning.

In the final vignette below, you will see how the therapist incorporates some of the IST themes into his work with the client, Rae.

Case Example

Rae is a 14-year-old female who was referred to therapy for anxiety, Obsessive Compulsive Disorder (OCD), and some recent self-injuring behaviors. Rae has an extensive trauma history, including being born addicted to the drugs her biological mother was actively using during her pregnancy. Additionally, Rae was subjected to physical abuse and neglect in her first three years of life before being placed permanently in the care of her paternal grandparents.

An IST-Trained Therapist's Intervention by "Bill"

Therapist: Hi, Rae! How was the week?

Rae: Not good. I started pinching and biting myself again. (*She begins nervously picking at the skin around her nails.*)

Therapist: Hmmmm okay, so any thoughts on what stood in the way of you being able to not self-injure this week like you had hoped?

Rae: Nope. The thoughts were just too big. I couldn't stop them.

Therapist: So sounds like we have some M1 stuff here to talk about, huh? I heard you say that the feelings of self-harm were just too big? Bigger than your willpower, Rae?

Rae: Exactly.

Therapist: Well, I can certainly understand that feeling of things feeling too big.

Therapist: So can you help me talk through this, Rae? Start with the first thought you can think of that crept up on you.

Rae: Well, I was in my Pre-Algebra class when this kid kept banging up against the back of my chair. He just kept doing it. And then I noticed that I had started picking at the skin around my nails.

Therapist: And then what happened?

Rae: I whispered, "Stop it!" to him.

Therapist: And then what did the kid do?

Rae: He banged up against my chair more. And harder.

Therapist: And then what thoughts came next? (*The therapist follows along these lines for a few more minutes to highlight the problem sequences for Rae.*)

Therapist: (*In a collaborative and curious tone*) But I find this interesting, Rae...some weeks you are bigger than the thoughts of self-injuring and you don't do it. But *this* week the thoughts were bigger than you. What do you think stood in the way of you being able to overpower the thoughts this week?

Rae: I don't know. I just feel like the thoughts kept coming, they wouldn't stop and no matter what I did, they just kept at me.

Therapist: So maybe we can talk about some ways to help calm those thoughts when they start poking at you. Do you want to practice some of the visualizations and mindfulness exercises we did last week with me now?

Rae: Okay. I'll try. If it might help.

In this vignette, we can see how the therapist opens up the session by asking a Negative Explanation Question and then building off of that with some work on Rae's thoughts and beliefs about what happened. The therapist challenged her narrative a bit and then highlighted the problem as embedded within a problem sequence. Lastly, he helped Rae practice some strategies to help with her M1 expressions in the hopes that these shifts might help her to be more successful in not self-injuring for the following week. This is a short sampling of some of the strategies an IST therapist might employ.

Key Takeaways

Integrative Systemic Therapy (IST) will always center on a few key concepts when using the model in playful interventions. The following are a few key elements to remember when working from an IST-informed lens:

- Since IST is a framework, those using it adhere to the notion that no one model of treatment is best. Rather, the framework allows for any number of strategies and interventions to be chosen based on the therapist's and client's assessment of the problem sequences and the areas that contribute to constraints.
- IST centers on the idea that there are three main parts to therapy—locating a problem in a problem sequence, finding possible solution sequences, and the possibility of constraints standing in the way of successful outcomes in treatment.
- IST adheres to a systemic view that shuns linear causality in favor of a more recursive view of how problems arise, and a preference for doing work within the context of family whenever possible. Thus, problems always occur within a problem *sequence*. Once the problem sequence is discovered and understood, the therapist can help clients move toward possible solution sequences. If the transition from problem to solution fails to go swimmingly, the therapist will then look for the possible *constraints* that serve as "roadblocks" to alleviating the problem. These constraints can also include factors related to things like culture or family organization. The framework provides therapists with a decision-making structure that suggests when they should borrow from other models of therapy.
- Therapists using an IST framework have many concepts that can be made into playful lessons for younger clients. These include the super-fun use of the Candy Jar Analogy, constraints (or orange-coned "roadblocks), or the "how" they think about things (levels of mind).

10   Gestalt Therapy

Model Background and Key Concepts

The word "gestalt" originates from the German term that means "complete" or "whole." Fritz Perls was the psychiatrist who developed this treatment model (Perls et al., 1951) in the 1940s and 1950s. One basic tenet of the model includes the notion that clients are best treated by looking at them as a "whole" that is made up of their physical body, their thoughts, and the emotions they experience. Integrating these parts is key to how clients look at themselves. Another central idea is that therapy should be more than just simply talking, but rather experiential exercises that help clients become more aware of themselves and what things are blocking change. The experiential component of Gestalt therapy makes it an especially fitting choice to draw from for playful interventions. Additionally, the Gestalt practicing therapist will provide an empathetic and non-judgmental space, while avoiding hierarchy or vibes of superiority, in the therapy room. This allows younger clients to not feel threatened by a parental or authoritarian impression from the therapist.

Playful Technique Ideas

"Wholeness"

As described above, the concept of being "whole" or "complete" is a central one in Gestalt Therapy. Therapists can come up with creative ways to help younger clients understand feeling complete. In addition to exploring how where in the physical body a child feels things, therapists will also want to explore clients' thoughts and internal representations of emotions.

One way to help the child visualize wholeness is by using a familiar, round food as a model. For example, therapists can have child clients cut out and color in a pizza, or cut a picture of one from a magazine. For teletherapy kid clients, it's easy to share screens and find a million different images online for the child to choose from. *Please note that this is an activity where cultural norms can be

DOI: 10.4324/9781003506072-11

easily considered by using something like Naan bread, pitas, cookies, or quesadillas if those foods are more commonly eaten in clients' families.

Next, therapists can help cut the "pizza" into triangular slices and label each with "parts" of the child that make them "whole." For remote clients, the whiteboard feature of the online platform can be used to draw and label the sections of the pizza. There are many angles to approach the parts from, so the following is one example of how to create and measure completeness in terms of relationships and roles:

> Label each part as who the child client is in relationships. For example, nine-year-old Brian's pizza might contain: friend, student, brother, son, and soccer player. Under each part, the therapist can help Brian brainstorm as to descriptors that best fit his role in each. For example, for the "friend" slice, Brian might choose: Peacemaker, funny one, loyal, kind, leader, and calmest one. The therapist can then expand the discussion to explore whether there are other things Brian needs to "complete" that piece of his pizza. For example, Brian might decide that "weak" areas include getting really annoyed by one particular kid in his friend group and wanting to make more friends outside of the ones he has since they are only from his soccer team. These can serve as goals for the client to explore, better understand, and design strategies for changing them.

Another, simpler variation for understanding completeness or wholeness is to draw a full circle on a piece of paper. Next, the therapist can make a tiny mark next to the full circle that symbolizes the very beginning of the curve of a circle. Throughout the session, the therapist can ask a lot of questions about what's going well in the client's life, and with each one, the therapist draws a bit more of the circle. Finally, the therapist leaves a tiny open dash of uncompleted circle and asks the client, "So what do you think is missing? What stuff would you like there to be more of, less of, or different that would help fill in this little blank spot and make your circle feel more complete?"

"Top Dog" and "Bottom Dog"

"Top Dog" and "Bottom Dog" are two common terms in Gestalt Therapy. They are particularly fun to introduce to kid clients, not only because they evoke a fun and familiar character and pet for many families (a dog) but also because they help break down a child's understanding of their "wholeness" into two distinct, and often opposing parts.

When a therapist notices a child client expressing two distinct, oppositional thoughts, perceptions, attitudes, or opinions, the therapist can label the two parts as Top Dog and Bottom Dog and encourage the child to explore these two parts and what they are all about. Some good starter questions might include:

- What motivates each one?
- On which occasions does each one show up?
- How do family members or friends react to each one?
- What is each one trying to say?
- What is each one trying to get you to do?
- What is each one trying to accomplish?

The Top Dog is generally explained as the one who needs things to be a certain way or embodies the role of what the client "should" do or think while often infiltrating societal or family rules or norms, while the Underdog is described as the one who is spontaneous, "acts out" or doesn't follow the rules, is rebellious, or gets in trouble.

To help kid clients better understand Top Dog and Bottom Dog, therapists can help the clients draw two dogs, one bigger, stronger and meaner, and the other can be smaller, skinnier, and more nervous and meek. Another helpful reminder activity for younger clients is to purchase a variety of dog stickers, and affix a few of the larger, meaner looking dogs to the top of the door or wall of the therapy room, while affixing the smaller, more fearful dogs at the bottom. The therapist can refer to these fixtures when appropriate and ask kid clients, "So which dog is taking over this situation—Top Dog or Bottom Dog?" or, "So, this issue with your mom and bedtime—do you think it's a job that should be handled by Top Dog or Bottom Dog?"

The "Here and Now"

One of the most powerful principles of Gestalt therapy is the focus of figuring out solutions in the moment or the "here and now." Using the guide of staying in the present, the therapist would try to help child clients stay in whatever the experience is that they are describing. So rather than just *talking* about how Mom is "unreasonable" and yells all the time, the therapist would ask the child to perhaps re-enact (similar to the Structural Therapy intervention described in Chapter 1) the situation with a focus on how each piece of it made the child *feel*. The following are some questions and statements that therapists can use to help keep discussions in the present, and on a visceral level:

- "What are you thinking right now?"
- "How are you feeling at this very moment?"
- "Stop for a minute—focus on what's in your mind at this very second."
- "Okay, so that's what Mom said *yesterday*, but tell me what you are feeling right now as you tell me about it *today*."
- "What's going on in your (head/heart/body) at this very instant?"

"What" and "How" questions are especially helpful in keeping clients in the here and now. Keeping child clients in the present is important for Gestalt-guided therapy, and it may also be appropriate to offer a simple explanation of *why* this is to kid clients who are developmentally able to understand it. The following is a template for a simple explanation of "staying present" from a therapist to her 15-year-old client "Cristian."

Cristian: My mother is totally unreasonable. She is so old-school and doesn't get how things are today. She like, screams at me for shit that *every* kid does and thinks I'm so freaking awful. But I'm not. She has *no* idea how good she's got it with me—I'm nowhere near as bad as all my friends are!

Therapist: Well, it sounds like you two have very different views on things here, huh?

Cristian: Yeah we do...

Therapist: So I know we talk a lot about how things have gone between you and Mom, but I want to ask you something about *right now.* I get that you are just generally really irritated and frustrated and maybe even mad about how Mom views things, but as you're telling me this—like, about how you think she's got it good because your friends are so much worse than you are—tell me what's going on inside your mind and your body as you say those words again. If you want to, repeat what you just said to me and try to focus on your thoughts and feelings *right now,* as you say it.

Cristian: Why do you want me to do that?

Therapist: Well, it's important to know the thoughts and feelings that have built up for a while from all the negative interactions with Mom this last year, but it's the thoughts and feelings right now, or in the moment that you're actually engaging with Mom that will really matter in how you respond to her. So if you're feeling really angry when Mom tells you she's really frustrated with you, you might say or do something different than what you'd say and do if you were feeling really hurt in that moment, right?

Cristian: (*Nods.*)

Therapist: So what if you and I role-play together now the next thing you think is going to happen with Mom and I'm going to ask you to stop at times and tell me exactly what you are thinking and feeling during our role-play. This way, we can guess how you will be feeling and what you will be thinking when the actual incident is happening next time and we can better plan for how you could handle it.

A playful addition to the verbal integration of the "here and now," therapists can laminate an index card with the words, "Right Now" and, "Then" on each side of the card. During conversations, especially with younger clients, the therapist can flip the card to one side or the other to have the client focus on thoughts or feelings in the present moment.

"I Statements"

The use of "I Statements" is a common intervention for many therapists who practice various different types of treatment. However, the real use of these as a therapeutic technique can be found first in Gestalt work. "Personal Responsibility" is also a foundational piece of clinical work for Gestalt-guided therapists that links well with the use of "I Statements."

Especially with younger clients, with whom therapists may be helping to build a foundational understanding of self, instilling the value of personal responsibility for thoughts and actions is paramount. One way to do this is by teaching younger clients about using "I statements." Using these statements in communication helps the child and/or family members focus on their *own* actions and feelings (of which they can be in control of), versus those of *others* (of which they cannot be in control of and will generally just be reactive to). The following are some playful ways for therapists to incorporate "I Statements" into therapeutic work:

- Therapists can begin the sentences for child clients with an exaggerated "I" (e.g., "So tell me how things went this week at home. Let's start with, 'I-I-I-I-I-I felt.......")
- Therapists can use the "fill in the blank" game, where therapists provide a series of questions for younger clients to answer, all beginning with "I." These can either be found ready-made online, or therapists can create their own worksheets and print out copies, email to teletherapy clients, or laminate and use with Dry Erase™ markers for multiple uses in sessions. Sample questions might include, "I don't like when…" or, "I feel angry when…" or, "I am happiest when…"
- For younger clients, therapists can use stuffed animals or other figurines around the office (or the child's room or home for teletherapy clients) to represent central family members or friends involved in whatever the issue at hand is. Therapists can control pushing forward the figurine that represents the client as a reminder to speak from the *client's* own perspective using "I" as the first word.
- The therapist can make a game out of using "I Statements" by first giving an example of the difference between, for example, the following two statements:

  - *"I feel so mad when my Mom yells at me."* (The *client* experiences and feels something).
  - *"My mom makes me so mad when she yells at me."* (The Mom *does* something—e.g., "*Makes* me so mad.")
    Then the therapist can offer statements that the child client gets to "reframe" as an I Statement. For example, the therapist might say, "My brother hates me so much, he literally can't stand when I'm around him and he's so mean to me." The kid client can then try to offer a variation of

the therapist's statement by saying, "I feel like my brother hates me when he's so mean to me and I feel like what he says to me means he can't even stand to have me around." This second, revamped statement leaves a lot more room for the therapist to explore things like how the kid client is interpreting the brother's actions, how his feelings in interactions with his brother cause him to say or do certain things, etc.

Guided Fantasy

The intention of Guided Fantasy is a bit like that of role-playing. Both allow the therapist to bring the client's issues and struggles, both past and current, to "life" in the therapy room. Guided fantasy can look much like the relaxation and visualization discussed in Chapter 8. However, Gestalt-inspired therapists might expand that visualization and imagery to fantasize about certain situations they might find themselves in and how they would handle those situations by putting themselves into different roles. Therapists can help guide kid clients into relaxed states where they are able to imagine situations that the therapists set up in great detail for them. There are several strategies that can serve as next step choices, so here are a couple of solid ones that I've used on numerous occasions with kid clients:

- Therapists can help clients shift back and forth between their own thoughts, feelings, and actions and those of the other person in the situation so that they can glean a better understanding of the full context of the situation and interaction.
- Therapists can help clients imagine a difficult scenario and then guide them into imagining a variety of different actions they could take, and ask them to express how they are thinking and feeling as they "experience" each one.

Through these imaginary exercises, clients may be able to explore thoughts, perceptions, and feelings in ways that they simply were unable to by just talking about situations in therapy. Discovering these more deeply rooted, here and now thoughts and feelings can give therapists more information that they can use to help arm their clients with better and more thorough strategies and coping skills.

The "Empty Chair"

The "Empty Chair" is arguably the most widely known and used technique from the Gestalt Therapy toolbox. Historically, it has been mainly used in group settings, but there are several adaptations that lend themselves well to the more intimate individual or family therapy setting as described below. I have personally used this over my entire career in working with kid and family cases with great success. The technique works well because it takes advantage of young clients' enjoyment of make-believe and their ripe imaginations. Coupled with the interactive and systemic nature of this activity, it is a solid choice for use with younger clients and/or their families.

The Empty Chair is somewhat of a role-playing activity, but rather than doing it with the therapist or another live person, the client interacts with an empty chair in the room that they will imagine a particular person sitting in. This allows the rehearsal of saying things, as well as the safety of not having the person really there during the activity. A playful addition to this exercise is to have the child select a stuffed animal, doll, or other figurine to sit in the empty chair to symbolize the person with whom they will be talking to.

The therapist then prompts the child to have a conversation with the empty chair "person" about either a recent interaction, asking them a difficult question, or expressing how something makes them feel. The therapist's role can be to listen carefully for patterns or other helpful information about the client's thoughts or perceptions, or to direct the client to switch seats with the other "person" if the therapist feels it would be helpful for the client to think about the other "person's" perspective. Since younger clients may not have a vast repertoire of words or appropriate ways of expressing things, the therapist may also serve as a sort of "coach" who can offer possible things to say or ways to address things.

Another possible use for the Empty Chair technique is for the "person" in the chair to be a certain part of the client. The "person" in the chair can represent a particular part of the child client—the "sad" part or the "frustrated" part. For example, the idea of "Top Dog" and "Bottom Dog" (discussed above) can be played out with kids in session. This would include child clients switching chairs to speak from each of those two parts of themselves.

Undoubtedly, the Empty Chair Technique has numerous uses for kid clients. The final Case Example for this chapter will include a more detailed look at how this technique appears in action.

Identification and Exaggeration

The concepts of identification and exaggeration are central to the Gestalt model. They are very fitting for playful interventions with young clients and/or their families.

IDENTIFICATION

Identification is when the therapist recognizes repeated, observable patterns or actions and calls the client out on this. Some common physical responses might include things like grimacing, slouching, closing eyes, picking at or shaking a part of the body, or other physical gestures. For example, if nine-year-old Micah is biting her nails and chewing the ends of her hair in a session where she is talking about being bullied at school, the therapist can say something like, "Micah, I'm noticing that you've been biting at your nails and hair today while we've been talking about how the other kids have been picking on you at school. Can we stop for a minute and give that biting and chewing a voice and let it say what it needs to say?" Micah might answer, "I'm scared of those other kids," and the therapist might reply, So let's give that biting and chewing a name that's fitting for the feeling behind it—how about if we name that biting and chewing 'scared of bullies?'"

The objective of identification is for the therapist to help clients identify the ways in which their physical body plays out the emotions inside. Creating awareness of these unintentional actions or movements in the body can assist kid clients in understanding the link between feelings and how their physical self "embodies" them.

EXAGGERATION

Exaggeration goes along nicely with the concept of identification. Once a therapist notes an action to clients and has them explore it, name it, and give it a "voice," the therapist may choose to have child clients repeat, add emphasis, or exaggerate the action. This is so that the therapist and client will have the opportunity to further explore the thoughts and feelings that accompany the body's movement. It is amazing how frequently clients have a "block" to the awareness between the two things—thoughts/feelings and the body's movement—that are often occurring simultaneously. It is an important lesson to kid clients as well, that there is an incredibly powerful connection between mind and body.

Another way I have used exaggeration in a powerful and playful way with kid clients is to bring certain noticed body movements into conversations that may be difficult. For instance, while working with a six-year-old (Ari) who tends to burrow under the pillows on the couch whenever difficult things are discussed in session, the therapist might say, "Okay Ari, we're going to talk about that incident at the bus stop last week so this might be a really good time to bury yourself *real* deep under those pillows, as deep as you can possibly go. In fact, let me throw this blanket on top of the pillows for extra hiding power." In addition to exaggerating Ari's burrowing behavior, the therapist has also made a light and playful "game" of the behavior that can have a name, a purpose, and a "voice." Ari will likely appreciate the therapist's understanding action and become more comfortable with identifying and recognizing it. He may be able to talk about the behavior more readily and freely, while learning the link between it and the feelings that accompany bus stop bullying.

Experience Influences Perception

An important core belief of Gestalt practicing therapists is that no one is able to be fully objective. Every person is influenced by their environment, their community, their social networks, the media, their family of origin, their religion, etc. Hence, individual clients come to the therapy room with their own, unique and biased "lens." Gestalt-informed therapists will want to remember to regard each clients' "truth" as true to *them,* without imparting their own experience-altered perceptions onto their clients.

A playful way to help younger clients understand that "experience influences perception" is to use my "bug lollipop" intervention. Therapists can order individually wrapped, bug lollipops online at a variety of outlets. The lollipops have either a dead cricket, scorpion, worm, or a few ants, etc. inside the translucent, colored confections. When presenting a child client and/or the family with one of these lollipops, the therapist can lead an exploration of how any one person's individual life experiences will come into play when deciding their reaction to thinking about eating the candy. So for instance, if a person lived in a country where bugs are consumed as part of their normal diet, that person would likely be delighted to tear open the wrapper and suck away. Conversely, if a person is deathly afraid of scorpions for example, that person will likely be horrified at the bug lollipop and decline to eat it or even be in the same space as it. In addition to the tangible "lesson" the bug lollipop activity can offer, most kid clients I've introduced this with have shrieked in shock and delight at something they generally never knew existed. *Please note the cautions in Chapter 14 on things to consider before using the bug lollipop activity with kid clients.

Self-Awareness

As in many models of treatment, Gestalt therapy values the focus on self-awareness. This is especially true of younger clients who may lack the life experience, have limited exposure to and feedback from others, and not be able to developmentally answer the question of, "Who Am I?" yet. Experiential exercises like the ones described in this chapter are all important to use when helping clients to increase self-awareness.

Creative arts are at the center of the Gestalt therapist's activities to aid clients in gaining awareness and understanding of themselves and interactions with and perceptions of others. Given that it is an experiential, hands-on model of treatment, it is especially suitable for use with kid clients and/or their families. Engaging children or families in activities like painting, drawing, coloring, sculpting, and body expression and movement can help to open up the pathways of understanding of awareness in ways that might not be achieved by sitting and talking alone. Therapists should be sure to have as artistically well-stocked therapy spaces as money and space allow to utilize the creative arts in kid and family sessions.

Case Example

Ten-year-old Brielle is brought to therapy by her mother for issues of "acting out" and "mouthing off" and "attitude." After the initial attempt at a family session intake, Brielle screamed at her mother to get out, told her she was just a "mean old witch" and refused to talk to the therapist with her mother present. The following is a snippet of the therapist's individual session with Brielle, utilizing Gestalt therapy techniques, and specifically the Empty Chair.

A Gestalt Therapist's Intervention by "Andrea"

Therapist: Hey, Brielle. So can you tell me a bit about not wanting your mother in the session with you today?

Brielle: I told you, she's a nasty, mean old witch. I'm not going to talk if she's in here.

Therapist: What do you think would happen if you talked with her in here with us?

Brielle: Ugh, she makes me so mad. She is so freaking mean and yells and like, I swear she *hates* me and wishes I was never even born.

Therapist: Hmmm…well that's a lot to carry around weighing on your shoulders. So I heard what you said about mom, but I'm really curious about how *you* are feeling right now as you're telling me all of this.

Brielle: I'm so freaking sick of her. I hate her back. (*Brielle is sitting cross-legged on the therapist's couch and she is rocking back and forth so her knees are bouncing up and down.*)

Therapist: I notice that your legs are really bouncing around over there, Brielle. Do your legs normally do that when you're really frustrated and talking about your mom?

Brielle: I don't know. Maybe. I didn't really notice.

Therapist: Well, sometimes our body plays out how we are feeling inside and we can find a link between the two. Can you try to really bounce those knees hard and fast right now for me? And let's keep talking about how you *feel* when you talk about, I don't know, let's say that…you think your mom wishes you were never born.

Brielle: (Knees bouncing in a pronounced manner). I mean, who the heck wishes your own kid was never born? What mom feels like that?

Therapist: Has your mom ever actually said that to you, or you just *think* that?

Brielle: She's never said it but I *know* she wishes that, I just *know* it.

Therapist: I'm sure you have reasons that you think that, Brielle. But I'd love to hear more about how you are feeling, *right now*, as you say those words again to me—I feel like my mother wishes I was never even born.

Brielle: Awful. Sad.

Therapist: Ahhhh, so if we had to pick a name for those bouncing knees then, I'm thinking it would be "Awful Sad," what do you think?

Brielle: Yeah, I guess.

Therapist: And if we gave those "Awful Sad" bouncing knees a voice right now and asked them what they wanted to say, what do you think they are trying to tell you bouncing around like that?

Brielle: That I'm really sad that my own mother hates me and wishes I was never born.

Therapist: And do you think those "Awful Sad" knees would want you to try to figure things out and fix things with mom?

Brielle: Why would I want a terrible person who doesn't even want her own kid in the room with me here?

Therapist: Good point. I want to ask you if you'd be willing to try something with me.

Brielle: (*Shrugs.*)

Therapist: Okay, so let's pretend your mom is sitting in this chair. (*The therapist drags an empty chair over to Brielle and sets it up across from where she is sitting*).

Brielle: (*Smirks.*) Hi, witch (*she says sarcastically*).

Therapist: If your mom were really sitting in this chair right now, in here with us, what would you want to say to her?

Brielle: I hate you! What kind of a mother hates her own child? You don't get me at all!

Therapist: (*Coaching a bit*). Wow, okay, a lot of anger there. Can we give the "Awful Sad" knees a chance to speak here too?

Brielle: (*Sighs audibly*). You know it freaking hurts my feelings, right? Can you imagine how it feels to be not wanted and hated so much by your own mother? I'm not a bad kid, and you are just so mean to me and honestly, you deserve my yelling and attitude for hating your own daughter, you sick witch!

Therapist: Whoa, okay, that's a lot of stuff. Good job. So now I hear anger, sadness, and some real attempts at trying to tell mom how you feel. That's good. I wonder if she knows all the things you've said so far...

Brielle: (*Shrugs*). Probably not. She's so stupid and in her own warped world.

From this point, the therapist has a lot of potential pathways to pursue with Brielle. The therapist uncovered Brielle's perception that her mother hates her and wishes she was never born which may not be the reality of the mom and can be further explored. The therapist could ask Brielle to switch to her mother's chair in the hopes of having them both better understand Brielle's perceptions of her mother and what she thinks her mother thinks and feels. The therapist could also choose to focus more on the feelings that punctuate each of Brielle's thoughts and disclosures.

Key Takeaways

Gestalt Therapy will always center on a few key concepts when using the model in playful interventions. The following are a few key elements to remember when working from a Gestalt-informed lens:

- One basic tenet of the model includes the notion that clients are best treated by looking at them as a "whole" that is made up of their physical body, their thoughts, and the emotions they experience. Integrating these parts is key to how clients look at themselves.
- Another central idea is that therapy should be more than just simply talking, but rather experiential exercises that help clients become more aware of themselves and what things are blocking change. The experiential component of Gestalt therapy makes it an especially fitting choice to draw from for playful interventions.
- Gestalt concepts like Top Dog/Bottom Dog and The Empty Chair lend themselves so well to playful interventions to use with younger clients.
- Gestalt-practicing therapists will strive to provide an empathetic and non-judgmental stance, while avoiding and airs of hierarchy or vibes of superiority in the therapy room. This allows younger clients to not feel threatened by a parental or authoritarian impression from the therapist.

11 Strengths-Based Therapy

Model Background and Key Concepts

Although the idea of looking at people via their strengths had its roots in the 1950s, the perspective used today is a version created by a psychologist (Donald Clifton) who was known as the father of Strengths-Based therapy (Buckingham & Clifton, 2001). Therapists who are informed by this perspective should also be well-versed in a variety of models of treatment, as Strengths-Based is simply a lens used to look at clients. From that lens, therapists can create highly individualized treatment plans and interventions for each client, pulling from as many resources as possible to help create client-generated solutions. Strengths-Based (much like IST in Chapter 9) differs from the other chapters in this book, as it is a *perspective* and *not* a model, with its main goal to help the client achieve a strong quality of life and well-being, rather than aiming at diagnosis or problem reduction per se.

One of the most important ways Strengths-Based work is desirable when working with younger clients, is that if therapists are able to involve the child's family in treatment, especially the parents or caregivers, it can teach the entire system a more positive, strengths-oriented approach at looking at themselves, each other, and interactions.

Playful Technique Ideas

Getting to Know You

The Strengths-Based lens encourages therapists to see and treat individual clients like experts on themselves, their lives, and their experiences. For this reason, it is important for therapists to get to know their clients before jumping into clinical work. Many models will call this process "joining." A Strengths-Based version of this will include an intentional focus on getting as much information as possible about who the client is, so that there is a more thorough understanding of how they show up in the world and more opportunities for finding areas and qualities of strength.

DOI: 10.4324/9781003506072-12

Open-ended questions are of course the preferred modality of inquiry here, especially for younger clients who may need more time for explaining and descriptions and storytelling if they have a limited vocabulary. Open-ended questions elicit more information and serve as a springboard for weaving stories about self, perceptions, and experiences.

Questions and technique pathways to get to know clients can vary greatly, and all are okay as long as they are successful in connecting with clients, getting to know who they are, and gathering information on strengths they already possess. The following are some playful ways for therapists to get to know their clients:

- Play the garbage can game with kids where the therapist and client take turns tossing wadded-up pieces of scrap paper or tissues into an empty garbage can. Whenever one of them "makes a basket," they are allowed to ask the other one a question. Questions can start from super simple and fun ones like, What's your favorite color?" or, "If you could have any animal in the world for a pet, which one would it be and why?" Progressively, therapists can move toward deeper, more probing questions like, "How do you think your friends at school think about you as a student?" or "Have you ever been left out of something your friends were doing and if so, how did you feel?"
- Therapists can purchase inexpensive "spinners" (see Chapter 14 for more details on this) that can be crafted to contain different sections or colors or question topic areas to be used as a playful "getting to know you" game.
- Therapists can trace the outline of a child client lying down on a large piece of paper. Then, they can collectively fill in all the areas of the outline with information. For example, drawing a red heart in the empty chest area might prompt the question of naming all the people and things a client loves. Another example is filling the empty head/brain area with common thoughts and fears that the client has.

Retelling Stories

The Strengths-Based perspective encourages the telling of difficult stories, interactions, or experiences with a focus on infusing them with a more strength and resilience focus. One of the ways to do this is by changing the way we talk about difficult occurrences with clients. For example, if a child client describes being the "victim" of being bullied at school, the therapist can add the word "survivor of" [bullying] in order to emphasize the client's coping and resilience, rather than on their powerlessness, maltreatment, and torment. Consider the following snippet of a conversation between the therapist and 12-year-old Angel, who has been bullied at school:

Therapist: So it was a tough week this week with those two older kids in your PE class, huh?

Angel: Yeah, they kept mocking me for being small and told me to go back to Kindergarten where I belong.

Therapist: Well, how'd you feel hearing that from them?

Angel: I hate being so small! But I can't help it! Everybody in my family is short and skinny. I hate that they pick on me and they push me into stuff and throw the ball really hard at me. They're always so mean to me.

Therapist: How are you handling these PE days?

Angel: I change into gym clothes in the bathroom before I go to PE so at least I don't have to deal with them alone in the locker room.

Therapist: Wow! Well *that* is pretty resourceful of you—what a smart idea!

Angel: Yeah, it makes it better but…I'm like, *traumatized* by it—I dread going to PE and I get stomachaches before class and I'm embarrassed because I know other kids hear them and probably think I'm a wimp.

Therapist: Well, maybe that's what *you* think, but honestly, I'm really amazed at how strong you are to "keep your cool" and just ignore them— that's really hard to do. Do you ever look at that way? And I'm also really impressed that you get through every week with them and still go on to do well in your classes and be a good friend to the kids other than those two. I don't think you're a wimp at all—in fact, I think you are an incredibly strong person who deals with a lot from them and you just refuse to let it "stick." You aren't a wimp, you are a very strong *survivor* of really uncalled for meanness by others who have nothing better to do.

*Please note, in addition to the Strengths-Based work, this therapist was doing with Angel, the parents (with the guidance and support of the therapist and client) were working with the school to discreetly notice and approach the bullying dynamic that was set up in Angel's PE class. Additionally, the therapist was careful to assess Angel's emotional stability, additional support system, and coping skills throughout their work together.

Identifying Strengths and Successes

Remembering that the Strengths-Based perspective centers on the notion that clients (and families) naturally have all they need to work with and draw from in terms of strengths and resources, identifying these strengths, successes, and "wins" is an important therapeutic endeavor.

A good way to start amassing the clients' strengths and successes is by simply asking questions. Listing these strengths and successes allows the therapist to revisit the list at a future date to help clients draw from for use in difficult or challenging situations. The following are some great beginning questions to use to pull out the positives with kid clients and/or their families:

- "Tell me some things that you are good at."
- "Tell me about a time when everybody in the family was getting along and having a good time."

- "What are some adjectives you/your friends/your teachers/your family would use to describe you?"
- "What are some nice things people have said about you?'
- "What are some of your accomplishments that you're most proud of?"
- "What do people like about you?"
- "In what ways are you strong?"
- "What are some things that everybody contributes in this family to make it a loving one?"

To make questions more playful, therapists can ask kid clients to do something fun as they answer each question. For an example, consider the following scenario between the therapist and six-year-old Mackenzie:

Therapist: So Mackenzie, I'm going to ask you to do something before I ask you each question, okay? I'm trying to figure out all the good stuff about you so we know what stuff we have to work with in trying to fix some of the things you are upset about in your life.

Mackenzie: Okay, like what?

Therapist: Well, let's try it! Mackenzie, I want you to stand up, walk over to the door, and stick this sticky note as high up on the door as you can reach. (*Therapist hands Mackenzie a bright yellow sticky note with the words, "Things I'm Good At," on it*). Oh yeah, *and* I want you to do it as *fast* as you can, okay? On the count of three—one—two—THREE!

Mackenzie: (*Running to the door and affixing the sticky high up on it.*) Okay, now what?

Therapist: Answer the question—what are you good at? (*Therapist writes each thing down on a separate sticky note as Mackenzie lists them*).

Mackenzie: I'm good at doing cartwheels—nobody else in my family can do it! I'm a really good pet mommy—I'm always the one who remembers to fill the cat's water bowl and change the kitty litter and feed the fish. I'm the best at spelling in my class I think. And my mom says I'm the nicest to my little brother, more than my sister and other brother are.

Therapist: Okay, so now I'd like you to take these stickies with all these great things about you and find places to stick them all over the room. (*Therapist has written "good speller" and "caring big sister" and "good pet caretaker" and "master cartwheeler" on the stickies*).

Therapist: Great job, Mackenzie! Hmmmm, do you think any of these things you're good at could help us with the problems you're having at school?

Mackenzie: What do you mean? How?

Therapist: Well, let's pick one—how about being a good cart-wheeler?

Mackenzie: Well, that's silly! How can doing cartwheels make those kids stop being mean and leaving me out?

Therapist: Well, if we are good at something, it might be appreciated if we offered to teach other people how to do that thing so they could be good at it too.

Mackenzie: I could teach *you* how to do cartwheels!

Therapist: I bet you could! But how about if you asked those kids tomorrow if they would like you to teach them to do a super-duper cartwheel?

Mackenzie: I don't know if they would want to learn...

Therapist: I guess we can't know unless we ask them, huh?

At the end of the session, the therapist has Mackenzie collect all her little stickies and take them home with her, with the instructions to stick them all over her full length mirror where she will look at them and read them every morning to remember some of the things she is good at and can pull from as resources.

Once strengths are identified, explored, and listed, therapists can then pull from them for use in future situations. Consider two of the easily accessed strengths that six-year-old Mackenzie listed above—good pet caretaker and nice big sister. Even at this basic level, from the very simplest responses, the therapist might be able to focus on Mackenzie's ability to care about others, not just with words, but by showing up with caring gestures and actions and build that strength and quality out to apply in other situations (like being a good and loyal friend). From there, the therapist could brainstorm with Mackenzie about what things that she could say or do that would be good friend efforts.

"Super Powers"

Another, more playful way to incorporate strengths finding into kid client sessions is to evoke the concepts of "super powers" into therapy. Most kid clients understand this concept and what it means, but if not, a short explanation is as follows:

Super Powers are kind of magical things that some people have or can do that are really important or special. For example, (grabbing a Rubic's Cube™ toy from the therapy room table and aligning all the colors of one side very quickly) I can complete one side in less than 10 seconds. That's kind of like a super power because not very many people can do that. Your mom being a mechanic is a super power because she can fix cars that have broken down. And *you* have the super power of being the peace maker and being the only one in your family that can stop your sisters from fighting.

Strengths-Based work with kid clients can include exploring what super powers the child has and then figuring out how and where they can be best used. To make this more playful, therapists can help kid clients create paper crowns that have their super powers listed on them and decorate them with sequins and stickers and glued on gems. The mother of a four-year-old client I worked with brought his crown down to wear every night at the dinner table to help him with manners and not having tantrums. She told him, "I know you and Doctor Lisa made this special crown with all your super powers in it and I bet this crown will help you conquer the dinner table tonight!"

"Drains" Activity

Everyone knows that no matter how strong and resilient we are, excessive "drains" in our lives can wear us down and detract from those strengths and resources. "Drains" can be things like not getting enough sleep, constant cycles of arguing with someone, stress and worry, or procrastination. Helping kid clients identify their drains and ways to reduce them can be key when looking to maximize their ability to draw from their strengths.

When I had an in-person practice, I used these tiny matching grocery carts for this activity. They were doll-house sized and I labeled one as "Drains" with a sticky note, and one as "Fill Ups." These carts may be difficult to replicate, but therapists can use any matching baskets, boxes, or other small containers for this activity. First, therapists can explain drains and give a few examples. Next, therapists can ask clients to identify the drains in their lives and either write each one down on a sticky note, or add a marble, small stone, or other objects to the drains container of choice. Now there is a "living" pile of drains that can be explored, discussed, and strategized about.

Along the way, therapists should look for ways to highlight strengths that may show up when discovering drains. For instance, if a kid client reports a drain of, "My mother always makes me spend so much time with my sick grandmother and do stuff for her," the therapist can call attention to the child being a compassionate and loyal grandchild who embodies selflessness in giving time to the grandmother when the child might rather be doing other things.

An adaptation for teletherapy kid clients is to share screen and pull up an image of an overflowing cup of milk, a pot of water that is boiling over on the stove, a battery with a flashing "low charge" warning, or a car broken down on the side of the road. Keeping this image up and central as a visual can help the conversation about drains, and overload, and breakdowns more meaningful.

Reframes of Strength

Sometimes, strengths are not as straightforward and as easily accessible as others might be. People are multifaceted, multilayered, and complex beings. Words and labels are powerful and carry social stigma and expectations. There are occasions where therapists can be useful in pulling things that might at first be viewed as negatives, problems, or weaknesses but are really more appropriate to view as strengths. Reframes of things as strengths is a skill that therapists can teach the kid and family clients they see for therapy. The following are some common labels and some more accurate reframes of them as strengths:

- "Too sensitive" = Demonstrates empathy
- "Mouthiness" = Struggling to find effective ways to accurately communicate or express
- "Talks over people and interrupts" = Eager to share and having difficulty being patient
- "Won't listen" = Persistent and determined
- "Lazy" = Needs more motivation
- "Stubborn" = Strong willed
- "Chaotic" = Overly flexible

The descriptors on the left are simply labels, most with a negative connotation. The list on the right, however, containsdescriptors that can be seen as positives or strengths as well, but they also leave openings for goal setting on how to better achieve them. These reframing activities can be helpful to include parents or caregivers on, especially if they contribute to the more negative labeling in the family.

"Context King"

When seeing kid clients and/or their families, there is a "character" I created that can help in incorporating Strengths-Based work into sessions. The strengths lens focuses on context as being paramount to working effectively with clients. Niemec (2018, p. 94) wrote, "Context is king," when referring to how therapists and clients must consider the setting and situation before using certain strengths. For example, being super organized and neat and tidy in one's own home may be seen as an annoyance or judgment if that person tries to use those strengths while at someone else's house. Likewise, a child client who is an eager and involved student whose efforts and motivation are greatly appreciated by the teacher may not be so welcome when the same child is asking questions during a moment of silence or the teacher's lunch break.

In response to the important theme of context, I created the "Context King," which is a small laminated magazine cutout of a goofy-looking king image with a handle-bar moustache and a shiny crown. If therapists cannot find something similar, they can just use the verbal concept of the "Context King" or don a paper crown to symbolize it. When kid clients bring up situations without recognizing the bigger context surrounding them, therapists can crack out the "Context King" crown or cutout and say, "Hmmm…I think we have other stuff to consider here." The case vignette at the end of the chapter will illustrate further how powerful the "Context King" can be in kid sessions.

"Toxic Positivity"

"Toxic Positivity" is most often heard as a cautionary opinion of the Strengths-Based perspective, in that critics describe it as focusing too much on positives and strengths that it doesn't leave any space for the genuine negative thoughts and feeling that people can naturally have.

In order to avoid toxic positivity in my sessions with kid clients, as well to use the term as a way to underscore a healthy way to look at problems and solutions, I incorporate this in work I do with children and families. First, therapists can explain to kid clients (who are developmentally mature enough to understand it) and their parents or guardians that there are two ways to feel better. One is to figure out the "bad stuff" and get rid of it, and the other is to find the positives and strengths and pile them up so high that they eventually choke out the bad stuff. I use the analogy of a few rogue weeds popping up in a beautiful garden that if left unchecked, will likely take over all the beautiful flowers. Do we want to pluck all the weeds out or do we want to keep planting and watering more and more beautiful flowers so they leave not even a millimeter of space or sun left for the weeds to grow?

Another helpful way to "hit home" the utility of building positives and strengths, while still leaving space for the natural occurrences like negativity, sadness, hurt feelings, or just having a "bad day" is by using toy cars, a roadway, and a breakdown lane. This can be achieved by either drawing a two-lane, meandering "road" on a piece of paper or by building one on the floor or table with small, plastic "bricks" or blocks (like Legos™), both with a narrow edge representing the breakdown lane. Little toy cars are ideal, but therapists can use any small objects in the office to depict the cars.

Using the cars to demonstrate, the therapist then explains that each person (or "car") can be traveling down the road merrily for miles and miles, noticing the beautiful scenery, waving at other drivers, chugging along on their way to their home, a restaurant, a friend's house, or a restaurant or other fun outing. Next, the therapist tells the client that sometimes there is a reason that the car needs to slow down and pull over in the breakdown lane. The car won't stay there very long, but the driver needs to take a break maybe, stretch, get a water out of the back seat, check on an engine light or other possible problem with the car. In extreme cases, maybe the driver needs to call for help or have a tow truck take the car in for service if it breaks down. So too are there times in life where we might have a tough day, need a little break, or need to pull over and ask for help.

Going forward, the therapist can refer to "the breakdown lane" when issues crop up for clients that render them in a more negative space. The therapist can then remind them that the breakdown lane is there for a reason, and it's okay to use it, and that we will soon be back on the road again. From there, therapists can strategize with clients about the resources, supports, and strengths they have as options to use if they find themselves in the breakdown lane.

Worksheets and Activities

A really helpful thing that the Strengths-Based perspective offers practicing therapists is a wealth of ready-made worksheets and activities online. There are innumerable sites that include sample questions, guides, and activities for therapists to use to keep a Strengths-Based focus in sessions. Although most are not specific to child clients, a creative therapist can easily craft more kid-friendly and playful versions of them. Given the Strengths-Based focus on creating highly individualized interventions that utilize the clients' expertise on themselves and their unique strengths, tweaking online resources to fit specific clients is desirable.

Therapists who wish to learn more about incorporating a Strengths-Based perspective in their traditional work can attend a training or workshop or watch online videos of different therapists using this lens in their work. This chapter offers my own clinical interventions for kids, clients, and/or their families based on the Strengths-Based perspective, but therapists can feel free to use their own creativity to concoct playful ways to get across the Strengths-Based messages.

Case Example

Fourteen-year-old Bhavya presents for therapy after struggling with anger and depression over constant frustration and fights with her twin sister. They share a room at home and the stress and fighting have made her dread even being in her room and she also expresses anger at her dad for not following through on the requests Bhavya makes about her sister being more respectful, responsible, and organized.

A Strengths-Based Therapist's Intervention by "Tom"

Bhavya: My stupid sister was at it again this week—she wore my favorite sweatshirt to school and got stains all over it and then just took it off and dumped it on my side of the room. She's such a slob and has like, *zero* remorse for *any* of it.

Therapist: More of the same then, huh?

Bhavya: Did you actually think it would have gotten any better?

Therapist: You never know. Change can happen. We *hope* it does anyway! We talked about some things last week, and I guess we should try to look at how we can use some of the strengths we identified a few weeks ago to help you out with this situation with your sister.

Bhavya: What? Like my strength of being patient? And organized? I'm definitely losing patience and my sister just won't allow me to be organized—she destroys *everything.*

Therapist: So Bhavya, I understand there are a lot of things that make you really angry about how your sister treats you and your stuff, and how upset you are that you think your dad only sees your sister's side, right?

Bhavya: Exactly. She takes my clothes without asking and we share a room and she leaves food and her garbage all around it, even on my side, and refuses to clean it up. And then my dad just yells at both of us and says that I take her stuff too and make messes so I should help clean it all. But that's just not true. He *knows* I'm the more mature and responsible one and when I tell her she's out of line and needs to clean up, she needs to listen to me and do it.

Therapist: So it's great that I heard you throw some of your strengths in there—you're mature and responsible and organized, right?

Bhavya: Definitely.

Therapist: And I'm guessing those are things your dad really appreciates about you?

Bhavya: Well, I *thought* he did.

Therapist: Oh, I imagine any parent would really value your maturity and responsibility and organization.

Bhavya: You would think!

Therapist: But I'm gonna pull out the "Context King" here (tossing the laminated king icon onto the couch next to Bhavya).

Bhavya: (*Laughs*). Oh *no,* not the Context King! You're not gonna wear the crown thing too, are you? (*Therapist smiles and shakes head*).

Therapist: I'm thinking that your dad does indeed appreciate those things about you in many ways. But I'm wondering if there's more context here we need to think about.

Bhavya: Like what?

Therapist: Well, maybe when it comes to your sister and the way she does things, he would like more flexibility and tolerance from you instead of more maturity and responsibility?

Bhavya: Probably. But that's not fair to me for her to have it her way.

Therapist: Perhaps so. But what if we reframe your sister's behaviors? You called her irresponsible and a slob, right?

Bhavya: (*Smiles and nods*).

Therapist: What if we looked at "irresponsible" more like "carefree?"

Bhavya: Sure. But either way, she takes my stuff without asking and ruins it.

Therapist: What about drains? Are there things that stress her out or get in her way of being motivated to pick up?

Bhavya: Yeah. She's bad with time management and she always waits until the last minute to do stuff and is always late taking a shower and packing her lunch every night.

Therapist: What do you think would happen if you bargained with her? You are obviously very patient and resourceful and organized—maybe she would appreciate some help from you?

Bhavya: Like what?

Therapist: Well, if you want her to pick up a bit in the room for example, what if you offered to pack her lunch for her one night while she showers if she agrees to pick up the room a bit? Do you think she's agree? And that might be a good start, right?

Once the therapist began to generate openings for possibility of change and using Bhavya's strengths in different ways, Bhavya agreed to have her sister join in on the sessions and then eventually allowed the dad to join and the family was able to strategize and agree on better roles for each of them to maintain for better functioning and less stress in the household. Other model work was used her, but the infusion of Strengths-Based concepts was helpful in instilling positivity in this family and their understanding of patterns and problems.

Key Takeaways

The Strengths-Based perspective will always center on a few key concepts when using the model in playful interventions. The following are a few key elements to remember when working from a Strengths-Based lens:

- Strengths-Based is a *perspective* and *not* a model. Therefore, therapists who are informed by this perspective should also be well-versed in a variety of models of treatment.
- This perspective has its main goal being to help the client achieve a strong quality of life and well-being, rather than aiming at diagnosis or problem reduction.
- One of the most important ways Strengths-Based work is desirable when working with younger clients, is that if therapists are able to involve the child's family in treatment, especially the parents or caregivers, it can teach the entire system a more positive, strengths-oriented approach at looking at themselves, each other, and interactions.
- This perspective has some wonderful concepts to build playful interventions from (e.g., the "Context King"). Additionally, the use of fun worksheets can offer Strengths-Based therapists another modality for treatment.

12 Psychodynamic Therapy

Model Background and Key Concepts

Psychodynamic therapy has its roots in the early, general works of people like Sigmund Freud, Erik Erikson, and others. According to the Center for Substance Abuse Treatment (1999), there are four major schools (Freudian, Ego Psychology, Object Relations, and Self Psychology) of thought and theory that culminated in the Psychodynamic model. The traditional model necessitated long-term treatment, but the more modern, briefer frameworks allow for more effective, short-term therapy.

Although infrequently used in the more modern, systemic therapy world of work with children and/or families, I chose to include some widely known, traditional notions from the model that are especially adaptable to work with kid clients. Some of the basic assumptions of this model are the power of the unconscious drives that humans have on their thoughts and actions, the importance of secure attachment, and the way symptoms of not having this show themselves in everyday behaviors. There is specialized training for therapists who wish to practice from this model, but the following concepts can be added into younger clients' treatment to give them another way to understand themselves, their motivations, and their behaviors.

Playful Technique Ideas

Unconscious Drives

Unlike many of the other models of therapy covered in this book, the Psychodynamic-informed therapist will include the idea of unconscious drives to their clinical work. Revealing deeply rooted unconscious thoughts can have a positive and powerful effect on things like mood, thoughts, and behaviors. In addition, uncovering these unconscious drives can help clients increase self-awareness and understanding of their feelings and actions. The following is one way to playfully explore the unconscious motivators with kid clients.

DOI: 10.4324/9781003506072-13

Free Association

One playful way to demonstrate the power of influence of the unconscious is in using a free association exercise. Additionally, kid clients enjoy this activity simply as a fun and interesting thing to do, so their general willingness and enjoyment of it is strong.

Therapists can start by having clients get comfortable and close their eyes. As per the traditional model, the client would ideally be lying down and facing away from the therapist so that the therapist wouldn't influence the client's thoughts or responses. However, for the informal use of this exercise, any comfortable position will work if lying down is not possible or desired.

Next, therapists can explain that they want the client to get as comfortable as possible, and to relax their mind, and not to think. Therapists then share that they will say a word and the client is just supposed to say the first word that comes to mind. There are no "rights" or "wrongs," and the exercise is just meant to free the pathway for unconscious thoughts to show up.

After the exercise is complete, the therapist can point out things like hesitation, unusual or uncommon choices in word responses, voice tone, or emphasis on words when responding to create avenues for further exploration of possible underlying motivations or "hidden" experiences that might unknowingly inform the client's thoughts or feelings. Consider the following snippet from a free association exercise with a 16-year-old client, Margot:

Therapist: Okay, are you all relaxed now, Margot? Are you ready to begin?
Margot: Yes.
Therapist: Okay. Relax, and just say the first word that comes to your mind. *Apple.*
Margot: Orange.
Therapist: Carrot.
Margot: Orange.
Therapist: Intrusive.
Margot: My sister.
Therapist: Strong.
Margot: Mom.
Therapist: Weak.
Margot: Babies.
Therapist: Love.
Margot: Romantic.
Therapist: Boyfriend.
Margot: Steve.
Therapist: Hooking up.
Margot: (Hesitation). Ummm....mad.
Therapist: Happy.
Margot: Sad.

Therapist: Vacation.
Margot: Stressful.
Therapist: Relationships.
Margot: Hard.

Please note that good judgment and care need to go into therapists' word choice for this activity with younger clients. For example, therapists should be mindful of potentially activating words with children who have experienced trauma, or the developmental appropriateness of using sexually suggestive terms. In Margot's case, her boyfriend had recently cheated on her, and although the two had been working through things together, the therapist suspected that some of Margot's depressive symptoms might be emanating from that difficult event.

After the exercise completion, the therapist offers the following dialogue that helps to open up some tense areas for Margot.

Therapist: So, Margot—I noticed some hesitation, and your voice wavered a bit when you responded to the word "hook up." Did you notice that?
Margot: Yeah.
Therapist: What do you think was behind that?
Margot: The word "hook up" made me think of Steve cheating on me.
Therapist: And...?
Margot: And then I got that sick, angry, hurt feeling in my stomach again.
Therapist: I also noticed that all your responses to words after that were kind of negative. *Sad, stressful, hard...*
Margot: Yeah, when I "remember" about what happened, it like, ruins my whole day. Even if Steve and I are getting along really good—it just kills my mood.
Therapist: Hmmm...so do you think the hurtful feelings that you have been trying hard to squash down and "forget" might be causing some of your depression that's cropped up recently?
Margot: probably.
Therapist: Well then, I'm glad we did this little exercise to start the session today because it seems that there is unconscious stuff about the Steve event that is playing out in how you think and feel right now. Is it okay if we talk some more about it today?
Margot: Yes, definitely. I need to let it out to someone. And Steve doesn't want to hear it—he's sorry and wishes it never happen and says he loves me and wants to move forward, not go back.

Free association exercises can clear "blocks" or suggest unconscious motivators that might need to be explored, and if nothing more, it can help clients relax and loosen up their minds in preparation for being more open to the rest of the therapy session.

Past vs. Present

In many of the more postmodern models of therapy, focus on the past is not as important as focus on the "here and now." However, the *past* is indeed important to the Psychodynamic-informed therapist in that past events can manifest themselves in what the client thinks and how the client acts in the *present*.

One of the ways I incorporate the acknowledgment of how the past can influence the present is by using a simple laminated index card with the word "Past" on one side, and the word "Present" on the other. During conversations with clients, therapists can pull out the card and flip it to one side or the other to prompt the client to look at the past and then the future. Consider the following segment of a session I had with a 16-year-old girl (who had just gotten her driver's license) and her mother, and how the use of the past-present connection was powerful:

Therapist: So it sounds like you two have just really been at odds with each other this week. I thought it seemed like it was a happy event for you both that Grace was getting her license. Tell me how things went off the rails since last week.

Grace: She just keeps nagging me and yelling at me for *nothing*. It's ridiculous how she doesn't trust me—and for *what?* I haven't done a single thing wrong with the car since I got my license and can go out driving alone.

Mom: You were late getting home last night, Grace, and you know that the state has a curfew for new drivers and so do we and you disregarded that!

Therapist: Why were you late, Grace?

Grace: I was like, *ten* minutes late, for God's sake.

Mom: *Ten* minutes late, just like you were going *ten* miles over the speed limit and you told me chill out and not get worked up over that??!! *Remember?*

Mom: (*To therapist*). She pushed the limits when I was teaching her to drive and she just always try to push a little more, go a little faster, stay out a little later.

Grace: That's not true! I told you I was ten minutes late because there was that construction crew out that night paving part of the road and I got held up.

Mom: You could have called me to let me know!

Grace: Ha! No I couldn't! I would've gotten in trouble for using my cell phone while I was driving! You are so unfair and just so dramatic.

After coaching Grace and her Mom through the conversation for a few more minutes, the therapist tried to elucidate how the past was creeping into the present without the two of them realizing it.

Therapist: Can I cut in here for a second? (*Both stop arguing and focus on the therapist, who then brings out the "past/present" index card and lays it on the table in front of them with the "past" side up*). So it seems to me that Grace's *past* behaviors, and Mom, your *past* experiences with her where you perceive her as always trying to get a little more, go a little faster, stay out a little later are informing your worries *now* (*Therapist flips the index card to the "present" side*) about what she is doing. Does that seem right?

Mom: Probably.

Therapist: And Grace, does that make sense to you that things from the *past* (*Therapist flips card back to "past" side*) are making Mom worry about what you might be doing *now*? (*Therapist flips card back to "present."*)

Grace: (*Nods*).

Therapist: So maybe what we need to do is separate the two things—past things that have happened and how things are going to go in the future, and talk about them separately and try not to have them stand so closely together?

Id, Ego, Superego

Id, ego, and superego are a classic hallmark of the Psychodynamic underpinnings. I have found them very useful and effective in helping kid clients understand the forces that are always interplaying within them.

First, therapists can explain that there are three "parts of mind" that are always interacting inside of us. The following are the general descriptions I use for each. Therapists can feel free to make them more complex, or pare them down based on the varying degrees of development of the individual clients they see.

ID (OR THE "DOG")

The id is the most basic, animal-instinct part of you. The id just wants what it wants, is interested in pleasure and immediate gratification. It is like the dog that jumps up on the table and slobbers down a chunk of the chicken dinner even though the family is yelling to it to get down and go away. The id takes what it desires and also makes choices to avoid pain. It is primitive and greedy and acts on impulse.

SUPEREGO (OR THE "SUPERHERO")

The superego is all values and conscience. It speaks from the place of the "right things to do" and is full of "oughts" and "shoulds." It encourages the ego to be strong and make the "right" decisions. It rallies against any questionable forces and fights the id. It is like the superhero perched on your shoulder, pointing fingers toward the correct choices, admonishing you if you even think about doing anything "bad."

EGO (OR THE "SELF"—YOU!)

The ego is the balance between the two—the id and the superego. It considers both sides, it embodies our wants and desires, but it also has a conscience. It remembers that there are social expectations and repercussions for choices and actions. It is the decision-maker, the one that governs what we ultimately do.

I will often use a dog and a superhero figurine to represent the id and superego, and write the child's name on a sticky note and use it for the ego. During discussions in session, therapists who are using these concepts can bring them into the conversation as necessary.

For example, let's take ten-year-old Mila who is sharing her frustrations with her therapist in session. She talks about feeling like the worst one in her dance class and feeling like she "sucks." She doesn't think she will make the dance team and wants to just quit the class completely to save herself from the agony. The therapist might choose to remind her that it sounds like her *id* is showing up a lot in dance—the one who tells her she sucks, the one that tells her to quit dance to avoid the pain of feeling bad anymore, and the one who doesn't want to face the other dancers who she thinks are better than she is. Further exploration could include how she might give her *superego* a voice and see what it has to say and then maybe working on strengthening her *ego* in order to make choices that are truly best for her.

Fixation and Regression

FIXATION

When people don't healthily work through things in their childhood, they may become "fixated" or stuck on that particular area. The fixation might become obsessive and the person's entire focus may be on that one thing. For example, let's take a nine-year-old client, Mary, who is so angry and frustrated that her mother seems to always give more attention to her younger sister. No matter what Mary seems to do, she feels like she just can't win her mother's attention. Mary becomes *fixated* on getting her mother's attention. Everything she does at school is with an eye toward impressing her mother. She is always trying to be the "best" daughter by helping out and cleaning up after herself. But still Mary is frantic that she is not getting enough attention.

REGRESSION

People can show "regression" or a return to an earlier stage of development when they become frustrated by being fixated on something that they can't adequately figure out. Regression is seen in Psychodynamic therapy as an unconscious defense mechanism (described in the next section below). Let's look at nine-year-old client, Mary, again. Mary has become so distressed by the situation and not being able to win her mother's attention that she re-gresses back to a more childlike stance. Instead of talking to her mother about how she feels (which is something a nine-year-old is completely able to do), she instead starts crawling into her mother's bed at night claiming her "tummy hurts" and starts trying to hold her mother's hand every time they go out.

There isn't really a playful way to introduce these concepts to child clients, except to use them as a way to psychoeducate parents or caregivers or child clients about the things that we sometimes do when we are frustrated. Normalizing and explaining it can be helpful, as can be giving alternatives to the regressive behavior that might work more successfully. The following is the language I have used with kid clients and their families:

- You know, there's this thing that happens sometimes when we get frustrated with something we can't figure out. We just keep focusing on it and might get obsessed with it and maybe that's all we even ever think about. And when that goes on for a while, then we can get so frustrated that we can't figure it out that we start to go back to our childlike ways of getting things. Have you ever seen a grown up ever get really angry and frustrated and have a kind of tantrum like they did when they were a kid? Sometimes that's what we do. So I'm wondering if this (e.g., acting out) behavior might be kind of like that?

Defense Mechanisms

According to Psychodynamic leaning therapists, defense mechanisms are things that help protect the ego or self. Life can be stressful for everyone at times, and sometimes the pressure can cause a person to want shrug off some of the anxiety that it can generate. That's where defense mechanisms kick in, to help diffuse the stress. All defense mechanisms are unconscious and all do things like twist, manipulate, misrepresent, or distort reality.

There are between 7 and 30 main defense mechanisms that various sources have described. I have chosen just a couple frequently seen ones in kid clients from the classical Psychodynamic model to focus on in this section (along with "regression" that was covered above in the last section).

PROJECTION

This defense mechanism focuses on a client's ascribing onto others their own un-acceptable feelings. For example, a seven-year-old client, Sam, is really annoyed by a kid who sits in front of him on the bus. He is so annoyed by the kid that he starts to think mean thoughts about him and fights the desire to be mean to him. Sam often bangs the seat back in front of him intentionally when he sits down to annoy the kid back. When the therapist asks about social relationships at school and on the bus, Sam describes the kid on the bus being mean and annoying and not liking Sam because he often turns around to look at him and says, "What?"

Sam is unconsciously holding onto dislike for the kid on the bus, but actually projects that dislike onto the kid on the bus and distorts the truth unintentionally by describing the kid as the one who doesn't like Sam, instead of the other way around.

This defense mechanism centers on explaining a distressing or emotionally charged occurrence in a logical way that doesn't allow for the truth of it to come out. For example, let's take our seven-year-old client, Sam, again. One day on the bus, a really cool kid that Sam likes and would like to be friends with decides to sit with the annoying kid in front of Sam. As the cool kid goes to sit down, Sam hops up and says, "Hey, you can sit with me if you want. You can have the window or aisle seat, I don't care which one I'm in!" The cool kid shoots Sam a weird look and retorts, "No thanks."

Sam's disappointment, hurt feelings, and rejection might cause him to "rationalize" the event in a manipulated way that doesn't reflect the real truth of what happened. Instead, Sam explains it this way to his therapist:

I didn't even really want that kid to sit with me anyway, I was just being nice. Plus, it was that dumb and annoying kid who sits in front of me who doesn't like me and wanted to get the cool kid to sit with him so it would him seem cooler. The cool kid just felt bad for him, what a loser.

Defense mechanisms occur often with kid clients and it can be beneficial to help them understand what they are and when people might be using them. A playful tool for kid clients on defense mechanisms is to create laminated cards with stock photos of different people glued one on each card. Underneath each photo, the therapist can print a scenario (see below for some examples). On the back of each card is the defense mechanism response. This is one way to help kids see what the defenses look like. The following are a couple of examples for defense mechanism cards:

RATIONALIZATION

Front: Joey gets a bad grade on a test.
Back: "The teacher is stupid and doesn't know how to teach us anything." (*Instead of Joey admitting he hadn't prepared for the test*).

ASCETICISM

Front: Ali is at the mall with her friends and has been dreaming all day of getting a burger and fries for lunch, but all of Ali's friends start whining about how they don't want to eat junk food and want to go order healthy salads.

Back: "Yeah, I feel *soooooooo* much better when I eat healthy stuff too. I have been dreaming about a big healthy salad for lunch like all day!" (instead of allowing herself to follow through on the meal that she really wants).

Attachment/Transference

Transference is an important concept for therapists to remember when working with kid clients, especially those who have had poor attachment to, disrupted attachment of, or abandonment by their primary attachment figures (e.g., parents, caregivers). A healthy and effective therapeutic relationship depends greatly on the navigation of this area.

Transference is when a kid client "transfers" onto the therapist things that have been unresolved with primary attachment figures. For example, if a (female) therapist is seeing a six-year-old boy who was removed from his mother's care, and then subsequently from his grandmother's care for incidents of abuse and neglect, the boy might act out his anger toward his mother and grandmother on the therapist in place of them, or create expectations of the therapist to fill the same role he expected of his mother and grandmother.

Since transference is an expected and naturally occurring phenomenon in the Psychodynamic model, it is important to predict it and face it head-on in therapy. One way for therapists to do this is to begin the first sessions with kid clients by defining roles of people in their lives. Clients can create lists or cards with things that each person is expected to do for them. For example, one child client might make a card for each of the following people—mother, brother, friend, teacher, therapist, neighbor. The following are some possible things to list for each one:

Mother: Love me, take care of me, hug me, cook for me, get me stuff I need, support me, buy me stuff, take care of me when I'm upset or sick

Brother: Split the chores with me, be nice to me, play with me

Friend: Be nice to me, stick up for me at school, play together, invite me over

Teacher: Teach me new stuff, make rules, help me understand stuff and answer my questions, make sure kids are nice to each other, be fair to everyone

Therapist: Listen to me, help me with my problems, help me figure things out, be a safe and trusted person to talk to, have good advice

Neighbor: Check in on me if my mom is late getting home, water our plants and feed our cat when we are away, bring us food when my mom is sick, be nice to our family

This allows the child to take inventory of the roles of each person and know what "lane" they will each stay in in order to better understand the difference in expectations for the various people in a child's life. During this activity, the hope is that the child will loosen the associations between therapist and mother, for example.

Case Example

Two brothers present for therapy, Jack is aged 10, and Jordan is aged 11. Their parents sent them for help with their constant fighting.

A Psychodynamic Therapist's Session by "Martin"

Therapist:	Hi guys. So who wants to go first? Tell me about what's been going on with you two.
Jack:	We fight all the time. Jordan gets me in trouble because he just always wants me to be the "bad kid."
Jordan:	He *is* a bad kid. He hits me all the time. And then mom or dad come in and they tell us not to fight and ask what happened and then I tell them and Jack gets in trouble because he hits me and hitting isn't allowed in our house. That's it.
Therapist:	Have you guys ever heard of id, ego, and superego? (*Both kids shake their heads*).
Therapist:	So we all have three parts of us that are always talking to each other, and they help us figure out what to do. So it sounds like being mad at your brother and hitting him is your *id* acting out. Our *ids* just impulsively lash out when they want something. I think your *id,* Jack, just wanted to hurt Jordan because you were mad at him. Does that make sense?
Jack:	Yup.
Therapist:	When does your *id* show up, Jordan?
Jordan:	(*Thinking*). Ummm…
Jack:	I got an *id* for Jordan! He calls me stupid. And he shoves the dog with his foot if the dog is lying on the floor in front of him if he wants to get by.
Therapist:	What do you think, Jordan? Are those examples of your *id* at work?
Jordan:	Yeah, I guess so.
Therapist:	Okay, so now we have the *superego.* And that sounds like your parents and the rules in your house. No fighting. No hitting. The *superego* is the rule follower, the superhero who points you in the right direction. Where else does *superego* show up in your house?
Jordan:	We're supposed to be in bed by 9 on school nights.
Jack:	We have to say please and thank you or our parents won't do stuff for us.
Jordan:	We have to finish homework before we can play video games.
Therapist:	Wow! That's a lot of *superego* around your house. Good stuff!
Therapist:	So Jack, now we see that your *id* tells you to hit Jordan when you're mad at him and your *superego* tells you no hitting in your house, so now you have this third thing called your *ego,* and that's the part that has to figure out what you are going to do next time you're feeling mad at Jordan.

The session carried on with the therapist exploring the three parts of minds and asking both Jack and Jordan what they each thought they should and shouldn't do when they were mad at each other. The therapist also helped generate new strategies for ways to navigate conflict between them.

Key Takeaways

Contextual Therapy will always center on a few key concepts when using the model in playful interventions. The following are a few key elements to remember when working from a contextually informed lens:

- One of the basic assumptions of this model is the power of the unconscious drives that humans have on their thoughts and actions. This is key to uncovering deep-seated issues that can contribute to and drive behaviors.
- Additionally, Psychodynamic-informed therapists focus on the importance of secure attachment, and the way symptoms of not having this show themselves in everyday behaviors.
- The Psychodynamic concepts of Free Association, Id/Ego/Superego, and defense mechanisms are especially fitting for fun and playful interventions for kid clients in helping them to understand the views that Psychodynamic therapists hold.

13 Best Practices

There are so many wonderful resources out there to help therapists design creative and artistic projects to use in their work with children. The previous chapters aimed at specific playful interventions based on a number of models that are widely used by systemic therapists. This chapter will center on some more general best practice tips for working with younger clients and/or their families.

Parent/Guardian Involvement

Since all of our younger clients will have some sort of parent or guardian or other caretaker as minor children, it is important to try to incorporate those folks in at least part of the therapy we do with our kid clients. Parents, guardians, and caretakers can learn from what they see therapists do in sessions and carry those things home with them where the child can benefit from more regular use of the strategies. Include parent(s) or caregivers in sessions whenever possible, or if not possible, share with them some of the playful ways you are working with the child so that they can replicate them at home. Modeling is key.

There may be many reasons why a parent or caregiver can't or won't come into therapy with their child. Some examples include:

- Time and schedule constraints
- Work
- Having other younger children to care for
- Having the mindset that the child is the "problem" and therefore the parent or guardian doesn't need to attend
- Worry about therapist's judgment of their care or parenting
- Feeling ashamed
- Disinterest
- Never having been in therapy before and wary about the experience
- Anger at the child
- Language barriers

DOI: 10.4324/9781003506072-14

Before starting a child-friendly practice, therapists can think of ways they might be able to alleviate some of the constraints to getting parents or caregivers into sessions (above). Examples might include having a policy where the parents or guardian has to come into the first session so that the therapist has the opportunity to assuage some of the caregivers' doubts and let them know how important their involvement is. Another idea is offering flexible hours for sessions to accommodate busy or working parents.

Cleanliness

Kid clients can be a bit messier than their older counterparts. Also, younger clients often lack the understanding of the importance of keeping a shared space clean and healthy. Some therapy space basics to consider:

- Chair or sofa covers that can be taken off and washed after spills, sneezes, dirty shoe marks, cracker crumbs, traces of glitter, or rogue marker lines leave their print.
- Pillows and stuffed animals that are washable.
- Disinfecting cleaning wipes or sprays (ideally child and environmentally safe products)
- A vacuum (especially if there is a sand tray or sand table in the room).
- Easy to wipe off plastic trays for use with activities that include things like markers, glue, or molding clay.
- A shower curtain or plastic mat to spread out on the floor for messier art projects.
- Hand sanitizer and tissues.
- Baskets or plastic bins for toys and art supplies that can be piled up or slipped under or behind chairs or couches in the room for extra space and easy storage.
- Posted (and enforced) any rules of clean up in the room.

Keeping some basic things in place in the office space will save therapists a lot of time and effort while still ensuring a fun and playful environment for kid clients.

Emotional Regulation

Developmentally, younger clients are more prone to being emotionally dysregulated. Any therapist who works with kids should have some training on and items in the office for helping a child regulate emotions.

Keep safe, touchable objects out for children to mindlessly play with when they are uncomfortable, having strong emotions, or just need sensory or tactile stimulation. Squishy balls, pin art impression toys, decorative wicker or grapevine balls, Silly Putty™, or a bowl of large marbles work well. Some therapists

I know have calming music playlists on their phones or big fluffy pillows for kid clients to hide under or wrap themselves around.

Mindfulness or breathing exercises and objects for distraction are good ideas. If a child client is prone to dysregulation, ask the parent/guardian if there are calming or comforting items from home that the child can bring into session. The "Calming Box" activity in the next chapter is another idea for a regulation tool to be stored for use in the therapy office.

Attention Deficit/ Older Kid Client Constraints

Certain kid clients may have reasons that they are unable to participate in some of the activities outlined in this book. Kids with attention issues may struggle to stay focused and on task in sessions. In this case, therapists need to ensure that sessions have a lot of activity and ability to shift gears as needed to enhance stimulation. Making playful games and challenges for taking turns, staying quiet, or counting internally to ten before speaking can help send a message of both acceptance of children's struggle and strategies to learn for self-control.

For younger kid clients, parent/guardian involvement or training is strongly recommended with treatment for attention issues because taking home the skills from therapy is an important part of the child developing better self-control. They may need help and prompts from parents/guardians at home to remember to practice the skills.

Therapists can have lots of things lying around for kids with attention issues to play with mindlessly while they talk or answer questions. Playing games like Candyland™ can help kids have something to play with the therapist while talking that is simply color recognition, so requires no computing or counting, etc.

Therapists should be liberal with breaks and changing up activities to keep kid clients' attention. Additionally, therapists can help distracted kids to refocus by instructing them to do a quick physical activity like jump up and down or do a little "happy dance." Another idea is to help them refocus by having them ground themselves on an object in the room, repeating a silly word, or still their bodies and put their eyes on the therapist's eyes and play the "staring game."

Older kid clients or teens, especially those who are less motivated for therapy, or are very driven by screens, may also have a more difficult time engaging in more traditional playful interventions. There are many resources online for incorporating electronic activities into therapy sessions with kids. However, I have personally found that so many "screens" kids are actually quite willing to engage in non-electronic activities if the therapist exudes enough playful energy and supplies interesting and pertinent activities.

Whatever therapists are comfortable with incorporating into their work with these clients will be helpful in making the therapy experience a more productive and enjoyable space.

Emotionally Dysregulated or "Shut Down"

Sometimes child clients, especially those who have struggled with emotional regulation or have a history of trauma, may become overly emotional or "shut down" in sessions. Therapists need to give themselves permission to "abandon" their therapeutic dance at times, and simply lean into their clients' needs at the time.

Spending a session on calming techniques, mindfulness exercises, breathing exercises, taking a break, or just doing nothing might sometimes be needed to help a child client work toward a stronger emotional space to do therapy.

Rules/Laws/Ethics

Let's start with the "rules" of the therapy space. Consider what things you want clients to know about safety and "rules" of therapy sessions and post colorfully on the wall as a reminder—include things like take turns, use inside voices, allotted clean-up times at the end of sessions, not leaving the room without asking permission, any safety rules, and the every session goals of "feeling safe" and "having fun."

Laws vary from state to state but all states have a mandated reporter requirement that necessitates that therapists be very mindful of any signs of neglect or abuse that might be present with a minor client. Make sure to have appropriate permissions and releases from parents or guardians for treatment and any contact with third parties that may need to collaborate with for the care of the child.

Ethics are important in all clinical work, but especially when working with minor clients. Be sure to update parents or guardians on interventions you are using so that everyone is on the same page. Ask about how they want you to handle things like what to do if they are late picking the child up from a session or if the child is particularly angry or upset.

Safety

Safety issues are especially important for therapists working with minor clients because they will often be present with the child without a parent or guardian.

- Keep child-safety outlet plugs in outlets.
- Lock up any fragile items.
- Make objects to be touched and played with easily accessible.
- Keep any items that are choking hazards, or games or toys with small parts away from small children that may be in your sessions.
- Keep sharp items somewhere out of reach that only the therapist can access. For example, not all children should be given free access to scissors or even sharpened pencils when they are angry or have issues with emotional dysregulation and might cause bodily harm.

- Ask parents or guardians first if the child can have anything to eat or drink in session, especially if the therapist has candy or other goodies in the office.
- Ask parents or guardians if the child has any allergies and be sure to get them to authorize an emergency contact in case the parent/guardian is unreachable.

Cultural Awareness/Inclusivity

Child clients (and their families of origin) each have their own distinct qualities and traits. Likewise, they each have a unique set of cultural and religious norms and values. Therapists should always be mindful of respecting and learning about the client's and the family's beliefs, experiences, goals, norms, and comfort level during the entire process of treatment. There are a number of ways that playful interventions too can ensure therapy will reflect cultural awareness and inclusivity for *all* children.

Therapists should be mindful of including items in their practice that are adaptable for various family types and cultural backgrounds. They can create an environment that is comfortable and inclusive for _every_ child. Dolls or other figurines should be of diverse styles, body types, and Crayola™ makes a line of crayons called, "Colors of the World," that represent a variety of skin tones. Another example would be to have Lego™ bricks in a variety of colors, not just the traditional "gendered" colors of blue or pink that often come in the more traditionally gendered sets.

Therapists should be careful of language, norms, and assumptions to ensure *all* kid clients feel understood. The use of non-gendered ("they" instead of "he" or "she") language should be used whenever possible. Terms like "mom" or "dad" can easily be replaced by "parent" or "person who cares for you."

Therapists should always ask first instead of assuming. For example, instead of saying, "So when you're at school," try asking first, "Do you go to school?" (in case the child is homeschooled). Likewise, instead of saying, "Oh, I'm so sorry to hear that your dad moved out, you must be sad," try asking, "How do you feel about your dad moving out?" (in case the child feels joy and relief that an angry and abusive father no longer lives in the home). Therapists want to be careful not to unintentionally send the message to kid clients that there is a certain feeling or response that is expected and "normal" for a given situation.

One of my favorite activities for getting to know a child client and/or their family is what I call simply, "Tell me about your family." After intake, I ask a bunch of questions, some serious and some silly. The following are a few of the questions I have used:

- Who is in your family?
- Where does your family live?
- Who lives with you?
- Who does the cooking in your family?

- What are some of your family's favorite meals?
- What are some of your family's rules?
- What are some of the things you or your family does that you don't think other people do?
- Do you have any pets?
- What are some things that your family does together?
- What holidays do you celebrate?

This activity is a low-key and casual way to begin to get to know the "lay of the land" in your kid client's life. The questions can be tailored to fit areas of religion, school, culture, values, or expectations. This also offers therapists the opportunity to learn about things they may not know a lot about or have personal experience with. For example, if a therapist celebrates Kwanzaa, and when asking the child about holidays the child reports that their family celebrates Hannukah, the therapist can say, "So tell me what Hannukah is like at your house. I don't celebrate that so I'd love to hear about the things that you do and what you believe."

It is so important to understand that in order for effective therapy to occur, clients and their families must feel comfortable and respected in the therapy setting. To the best of their ability, therapists should make their therapeutic environment and experience as welcoming, comfortable, and inclusive as possible for *every* client.

Competence

Therapists should be mindful of not practicing beyond the level of their competence. In fact, most professional Codes of Ethics contain clauses on this. If there are concerns that the effectiveness of your treatment has not been strong, or that there are more serious concerns about the child's level of trauma or diagnosis, keep the contact information for a local certified play therapist (CPT) and other specialists handy for referrals if need be.

Therapists who feel stagnant or stuck in their work with kids can search the internet for playful therapy resources, look up some online videos, or take a continuing education (CE) training on art therapy or play therapy for ideas to incorporate into their practices.

Teletherapy

Since the Pandemic, more research, resources, and guides have become available to therapists working remotely with kid clients and/or their families. Therapists need to ensure they are well trained/versed in best practices for assessment and treatment of this population in an online format. Teletherapy is not the most appropriate treatment for all child clients and/or their families. However, if teletherapy is assessed as being an appropriate modality of treatment for clients, many of the model-based interventions in the book can be easily adapted for the remote context.

A "plus" when doing teletherapy with kids is that they are usually in their own home, bedroom, or other familiar spaces. This can be a comfortable space for them, filled with their favorite pets, toys, or stuffed animals. Therapists have an inside view of the child's home environment and can ask about their setting. Their favorite things and props and toys are readily available to use with therapeutic games and interventions.

When working with child clients via teletherapy, I like to send ("snail mail") a brightly colored and decorated padded manila envelope to the child's home before we meet if that is agreeable to the parent/guardian. Inside of the envelope, I include various different "starter" supplies to use in therapy. I send a few sheets of printed paper or cardstock, some tool-shaped (e.g., hammer, wrench) paper cutouts (these can be ordered online or drawn on a piece of paper for the child to cut out), stickers, a package of colorful fun-shaped sticky notes, markers or mini glitter pens, and a few sheets of peel-off laminate. The child can be directed by the therapist at their first meeting to fold their selected piece of paper in half, and to staple the sides closed. Then, about an inch down from the top edge, the child will cut an oval shape in the center of the paper. This makes the arched handle to carry the "tool kit" they've just made. Children can personalize their "tool kit" with their name or some stickers. Each time a strategy, reflection, cognitive reframe, or helpful affirmation is discovered, the child can write it on one of the tool-shaped cutouts and slip it into the toolkit for use later. Parents and caregivers can add "tools" to the toolkit at home as well. The toolkit can be an activity for in-session kid clients as well, and the kit can go back and forth with the child from home and therapy to maximize additions to the kit.

Not only do children enjoy getting a surprise package in the mail, but they also love opening it with the therapist and talking about how to use the items inside. This is a great way to playfully "join" with kid clients and begin the therapeutic process in an enjoyable way.

Simplicity

Remember that although there is a wonderful array of therapeutic toys and games out there, the most simple and inexpensive items can completely suffice for doing effective playful therapy. I was challenged early in my career with being stuck in the only empty room available to do therapy with kids and families. There were countless sessions where I was able to engage children and do effective therapy with only some pencils, pens, paper, and sticky notes. Chapter 11 contains many interventions that require little or no preparation and items that can be found inexpensively or already lying around in the office.

Much like the old adage that one buys a gift for a child, and the child enjoys the wrapping paper and the bow more than the gift itself, so too are children often fans of the simplest fun. Taking a walk outside to collect leaves or rocks to paint, role-playing, drawing, or simple mindfulness exercises are free and available and great foundational pieces to a playful therapeutic experience.

Self-care

Playful therapy with younger clients can be draining and therapists should be mindful of the possibility of burnout when working with kid clients and/or their families. Many years ago, my practice somehow found itself filled on Saturday mornings and early afternoons with five back-to-back, under age seven boys with behavioral or attention issues. After several weeks, I noticed myself feeling more exhausted at the end of each Saturday and realized how much extra effort I had been putting into those kid sessions in order to keep them focused, engaged, and making changes. The therapy was very successful, but it came at a "price tag" for me. From then on, when I took on new clients, I layered adult clients or couples in between child sessions to keep my energy up. This was a really important and helpful decision for me that enabled my ability to keep working effectively with younger clients in a playful and energetic way.

14 General Interventions

The previous chapters in the book focused on specific models or frameworks to draw playful interventions in order to achieve more productive sessions and successful outcomes with kid clients and/or their families. The following is a list of some non-model-specific, playful interventions that can be used with kid clients and/or their families to make the therapy process more relevant, understandable, and enjoyable for them. This is *key* for successful work with our younger clients.

Many of the general, playful interventions require little or no expense or supplies. Below, the general interventions are divided into three sections—those with no cost or supplies needed, some with minimal cost or supplies needed, and those that require particular items or purchases.

No Cost or Supplies Needed

Mindfulness Games

The practice of "mindfulness" can be very important for young clients, especially those with anxiety or attention issues. Mindfulness games are hands-on, also of particular preference to kid clients. Therapists can start by having the child lie on the floor or couch, and the therapist can join them in this activity as well. For teletherapy clients, therapists and clients can lie on a couch, a bed, or a floor, and angle the camera to be able to still make facial contact. Have the child select an object—almost any object will do—and place it on their stomach. The therapist can do the same if they wish to model the activity for the client. The idea is to calm breathing so that the object moves less, more slowly on the client's stomach. The therapist can help guide clients toward thoughts that help calm breathing and make the object more still.

Analogies Games

Analogies are a comparison between two things and are a great way to help children separate themselves from the problem. Chapter 6 (Solution-Focused Brief Therapy) explores externalization as one way to achieve this separation.

DOI: 10.4324/9781003506072-15

So how do therapists help externalize children from their problems using analogies? Ideally, they will have a bit of creativity, but the easiest way to describe the child's issues or situation is to label it as something else. The following are some examples of how to use analogies to separate seven-year-old Casey from her social anxiety and angry outbursts at school:

- "The anxiety seems like a big ocean wave that you just have to turn your back to and let it take hold for a bit until it carries you to the shore."
- "It's kind of like when you're at the doctor's office and you're going to get a shot and you just dread it so much but then the doctor does it quick and it's over and you feel relieved."
- "It reminds me of the sun when a cloud floats across it, temporarily dimming its brightness, but behind those clouds is still a bright and shining sun."
- "Everybody has anger—it's like our own big Pitbull dog. It is a wonderful, loving pet, but sometimes it gets worked up and aggressive, especially when it's trying to protect us. We can have the Pitbull, but it's our responsibility to keep it on a leash and walk it away or cage it up if it's getting out of control."

Imagery or Visualization Games

Therapists can help clients (in person or online) close their eyes and imagine situations going better or approaching them in a different way. So, for example, if a child client expressed social anxiety at school, the therapist could help them relax and visualize getting up in the morning, feeling and acting confidently on the bus, and smiling and engaging with classmates. This can help them gain confidence, practice, and visualize things going differently than they may have gone in the past.

Imagery can also be used as a calming and distracting tool for children that suffer from anxiety. Guided imagery of a beach or amusement park scene can be relaxing and comforting. A child can then use this strategy on their own when stressful or anxiety-producing events occur. Imagery can be adapted to include the child's own personal preferences, cultural themes, family events, etc.

Beginning and Ending "Glimmers"

The term "glimmers" was created by a therapist who treats complex trauma and wrote a book called, *The Polyvagal Theory in Therapy* (Dana, 2018). She refers to "glimmers" as the moments when people feel in a space of calmness and regulation. This signals our central nervous system to relax and feel safe. In essence, "glimmers" are the opposite of the more widely recognized term, "triggers."

Helping younger clients to focus on the glimmers in their lives instead of on the triggers can help in several ways. First, like in the Chapter 7 discussion of "problem talk," it is easy to slip into worries and issues in favor of looking at positives and "exceptions" to the issues. Beginning and ending each session with therapist and client listing glimmers for the day or week is a good habit to practice. Therapists can send clients home with one particular glimmer to focus on and think about during the week to help them get through tougher times they may encounter.

Calm the Body and Mind Games

Relaxing the body and mind may be a necessary task before being able to effectively work with some kid clients, especially those with anxiety or hyperactivity issues. Breathing exercises, progressive muscle relaxation, and targeted sensation focus are great ways to help a client calm the body and mind. They can be used at the beginning of a session for optimal presentation for therapy, at the end of therapy to send clients off in a good space, or during sessions when things like anxiety or triggering occurs in order to return to baseline. Not only are these strategies helpful in sessions, but can also be learned "habits" that clients can use on their own outside of sessions.

Garbage Can Questions

The essence of doing therapy often includes asking questions. There are several ways that therapists can make asking questions playful, and one of my favorite strategies is the "garbage can questions" activity.

The therapist starts by taking a tissue, a scrap piece of paper, or a sticky note and balling it up. Next, the therapist tells the kid client that they will take turns "shooting baskets" into the garbage can. Each time they make a basket, they get to ask the other one a question. Not only do kids find this a fun activity, but it also allows the therapist to stay in control of keeping the playful environment therapeutic.

A variation of this game is for therapists to purchase (online or at an early education store) a blank "spinner" that can be personalized with numbers or sections or colors to represent types of questions. Clients can spin and whatever they land on has a type of questions to answer. Ideas might be categories like "things about me," "wishes," or "family relationships." Laminating the surface area of the spinner allows for reuse with different sections and question topic areas for different clients.

Externalization "Monster" Activities

As is discussed in Chapter 6, the idea of externalization is particularly helpful with younger clients so they don't end up feeling that they "are" the problem. Also discussed in that chapter is the externalization "monster" activity. This both helps children understand that they are *separate* from the problem and sets up the mindset that they can be in control of their "monsters."

Body Movement/Exercise Games

Younger clients often have a difficult time simply sitting still and talking. Fitting body movement or exercise into therapy can be beneficial to keeping kid clients' attention. Peppering physical activity into meetings is a good strategy to use with younger clients. Therapists can use the most simple, "Simon Says" games or "time out stretches" or "shake it off dances" in session. Additionally, they can incorporate bursts of energy into time together, like running down the hallway and back, or timing the child picking up all the toys from the floor.

Holding sessions outside of the building or while going for a walk with the client can be helpful strategies as well; however, there are additional ethical and safety concerns here. The permission of parent or guardian is required, and discussions about how seeing people outside of session will be handled are necessary. The child's ability to pay attention, follow directions, and not "bolt" are also things to consider.

One of my most successful child cases was with a 12-year-old girl who presented with depression and bullying at school due to being severely overweight and having a binge eating disorder. She was desperate to lose weight, learn better eating habits, and improve her self-esteem. She reported finding exercise boring and "dreadful" and used binging as a way to feel with her feelings of sadness or shame. We created our (teletherapy) plan to include sessions twice a week. During the sessions, the client would either go walking with her headphones on for our sessions or we would take turn challenging each other to an exercise between conversations. For example, she would choose ten leg lifts on both sides, and I might choose five sit-ups and five waist twists. We listed her likes/dislikes in foods and searched together online to create easy meal plans. We talked about self-esteem and body image and employed a number other therapeutic techniques and topic areas in her treatment. However, at the end of the therapy, the client reported that being able to use the therapy time to find motivation, more positive self-esteem, hopefulness, and a new belief that listening to her body more, eating healthier and exercise could be "almost" kind of fun.

Minimal Cost or Supplies Needed

Red Light/Green Light

Another playful way for kid clients and/or their families to practice boundaries, taking turns, and communication is using the red light/green light game in session. If the game is helpful to the client/family, the therapist can send them home with the craft, or you can use a laminated one that stays in the office. First, therapists will need to cut out two octagons of the same size, one out of green and one out of red construction paper. A large popsicle stick gets inserted between the two pieces of paper and the octagons are either glued or stapled together around the popsicle stick. Have the child client print "stop" on the red side and "go" on the green side. Another variation of this is to cut out one rectangle and color three circles (to represent "lights") in red, green, and yellow.

Next, the therapist explains that when a client or family member is feeling uncomfortable or angry or upset by a conversation or question, they can grab the craft and hold up the red light sign or point to the red "light" on the rectangle traffic light sign. Likewise, the green light sign can be used to signal when the questions and conversations are comfortable, helpful, and okay to pursue. With the traffic light craft, the yellow light can be used to signal the "getting dangerous" or "proceed with caution" or "slow down" feeling that might come between the red and green lights.

Laminating these crafts allows the therapist to use over and over in sessions, and quick ones can be created in the session to send home with the child if the therapist feels the tool would be helpful at home as well. For older kid clients who may not want to use the crafted red light/green light, the therapist can use the verbal expression of this in sessions. For example, the therapist might say, "Hey, I notice you're getting a little quiet—are we in a yellow light zone here?" or, "Okay, I hear you telling me angrily that you're not going to talk about this today. I'm guessing my questions were red light ones. Is there anything I can do or say differently that would make my question a green light one?"

The "Miracle Question" or Magic Wand Question

Chapter 7 centers on the Solution Focused concept of "the miracle question." For younger clients, I like to use the "magic wand question" as a more playful alternative of the miracle question. Kids clients can wave around either a real magic wand prop in the therapy office, or find something to represent a magic wand in their home (for teletherapy clients), or simply grab a pencil, a stick, or a highlighter. The therapist then asks the child if they were to wave the magic wand and their life became perfect overnight, what would have changed? What would their life look like? This elicits a list of goals very quickly for the client and therapist, as well as instills a sense of hopefulness and focus on change.

Journaling Activities

Journaling is a common practice in many therapeutic settings and there is a fair bit of evidence that it can be an effective tool to incorporate into clinical work. Sohol et al. (2022) conducted a research review and meta-analysis of journaling as a tool for managing mental illness. Although their findings were not conclusive, the benefits of use and very low risk of adverse effects were enough support for them to recommend use of journaling as an adjunct therapy to compliment other evidence-based management.

The problem with journaling with kid clients is that it is not a good strategy for *all* kids. Some clients may view journaling as a writing task and will hate to do it. Others may feel like it's "homework" and not want to do anything similar to what they have to do at school. Therapists can consider journaling as a *possible* intervention, but only after creating the most playful and fun ways to approach it.

Journals can be created most simply by just stapling together some blank sheets of paper and decorating with stickers or stamps. Therapists can also order fairly inexpensive bulk packs of thin journals online, or but a bunch of single-subject notebooks to give out to kid clients. Buying notebooks (and other creative play, art, craft, and office supplies) is cheapest right after the back-to-school rush after the end of the "summer."

The therapist (or family members) can create prompts and write them in the journal, the child client can choose to write about whatever they decide over the week's occurrences, or the journal can be specifically for something like "dumping anger" or writing letters about feelings to someone that the child won't ever talk to. Journals should have no "rules" that would make it feel like an assignment. Therapists can start the journal for a kid client by writing an affirming statement on the first page and drawing items around it that symbolize it— rainbows, smiles, or barbells to signify strength. Another helpful use of journals is to have clients read journal entries from the beginning of therapy to see how much change and progress have been made.

Affirmation Take-Homes

This may be one of the most personalized and effective strategies I have ever used with kid and teen clients, and is especially well suited for teletherapy sessions. Therapists and kids can use a search engine together to look up things like "affirmations for self-esteem" or "inspirational quotes on letting go of anger" (whatever the kid client's presenting issues are). They should choose pictures or quotes that most resonate with and make sense to the kid client. Then, the memes or quotes or photos can be printed out and laminated to take home as reminders of powerful messages or guides. Clients can put them in their school lockers, backpacks, notebooks, or bedside tables or dressers. An added touch is to add a tiny bit of magnetic strip on the back of the printed, laminated quote so that it can attach to a metal surface like a locker, a mirror, or the refrigerator. A big roll of peel-off-backing magnetic strip can be purchased inexpensively online or at any craft, office supply, or retail chain store.

Memory Aids

Yet another great use for brightly colored sticky notes is to work in session with younger clients to create a sticky note for each task they need to remember or complete at home. The sticky notes can then be affixed to places in the house that will serve as prompts for things that need to be done in those areas. For example, I was once working with a family that had "very forgetful" nine-year-old twins. Each twin got a small stack of their own chosen color of sticky note and specific tasks were written on each one. The following session, one of the twins shared that when he pulled his packed lunch for school out of the refrigerator, he saw the sticky note on his lunchbox that stated, "Put breakfast dishes in the dishwasher." He also shared that the reason he remembered to take his lunch from the refrigerator was because there was a sticky note reminding him to do so on the tube of toothpaste that he used to brush his teeth, and so on.

Worksheets

There are so many wonderful child therapists and agencies that create worksheets for kid clients on a myriad of topic areas. A simple online search will yield so many sites that offer free, downloadable (for email to teletherapy clients), or printable (for in-person clients) worksheets. Therapists can keep copies of different worksheets in labeled folders for a variety of issues like anxiety, self-esteem, sibling fighting, depression, and grief and loss. Therapists can also laminate a copy of each worksheet to be completed by the child client in session with Dry Erase™ or other brand of erasable markers, then wipe off for use with the next client.

Drawing/Coloring

Drawing and coloring are enjoyable activities for most children and should be a staple in every therapy office. Drawing and coloring allow younger clients to express non-verbally before they have a mature vocabulary. It can also be a mindless activity to do while talking to a therapist about difficult or stressful topics. Additionally, therapists can offer prompts for independent or collaborative drawing or coloring that direct the content toward a particular area.

Emotions Emojis

Adults often have enough life experience to understand a wide assortment of emotions and the various ways that they can be expressed by people. Child clients may not fully understand the range of common emotions and what they are, where they come from, and different ways of managing them. This can contribute to difficulties they might have in expressing their own emotions or understanding the way that others might exhibit theirs.

Therapists can print out a number of versions online, or order colorful posters from companies on the internet that display a huge range of possible emotions with human faces expressing those emotions on them. For a less expensive alternative, therapists can create their own poster of faces with different expressions that symbolize any number of emotions. Common emotions to explore with kid clients might be sadness, happiness, anger, jealousy, hurt, depression, fear, frustration, and hopelessness.

Magazine Collage Activity

Although most offices have abandoned print versions of waiting room magazines, it is easy for therapists to create a stack of store flyers and catalogues, and ask family members or office mates to donate their old print magazines for your child-friendly cause. Additionally, places like bigger medical offices, dentists, and libraries are more than happy to share their old copies when they change out magazines in their facilities each month. Collages are just a bunch of cut-out magazine words or pictures that are glued onto a single piece of paper. Therapists can help child clients pick a "theme" for this project and help them create a collage to go home with. For example, a therapist might help the child cut out words and pictures of things that make the child feel happy and calm. This collage can then be hung next to their bed to look at and calm them if they experience nighttime anxiety.

Require Specific Items

The Soothing Box

This is also sometimes called a "calming" or "anxiety" box, and is a really simple thing to create with young clients, especially for those with anxiety disorders. Recently, one of my graduate Marriage and Family Therapy (MFT) students came up to me after a presentation and told me tearfully that her childhood therapist had done such a box with her as she dealt with her parents' divorce, the loss of her grandmother, and a geographical move. She shared that even as a 30-something adult now, she still had her box and it was something that she cherished and gave her great comfort as a young person.

The concept is super simple. Get a box, any box. Cardboard shoe boxes or craft store wooden, paintable boxes are great choices, but anything will do. I once had a creative little child client who wanted his soothing box to be inside of his favorite empty cereal box since it was something that made him happy and he was only allowed to buy this cereal on very special occasions.

Therapists then work with clients to fill the box with items that calm or sooth them, or make them feel better. Mementos of happy times (like a pressed penny from a family outing to a big amusement park or the stub of a movie theatre ticket), or favorite items (like a small stuffed animal or beaded bracelet), or people that love and support the child (like photos of a stepparent, teacher, grandfather, or best friend) can be included. Printed-out affirmations or drawings or cutouts of favorite foods are also fun inclusions. One client I had put in a lock of her baby hair that her mother had kept, and an orange dog collar with the name

"Rocky" emblazoned on it from a beloved pet that had passed away. Whatever the items, the client should choose things that make them feel better.

Painted Rocks

Many people have seen the trendy practice of leaving inspirational messages on painted rocks in random places for others to find. Along this same vein, therapists can help child clients create painted, flat rocks that have words or quotes or other pictures on them that are soothing or empowering to them. Painting the rocks will take part of two sessions, given that one side must dry before the other side can be painted. Conversely, therapists can paint a bunch of rocks on their own and have them ready to be personalized by clients. To ensure the rocks are waterproof, therapists will have to take the rocks outside and spray them with a shellac coating before they will be ready for the client to take home. These rocks can be kept at home or in a desk or locker or school, or even be created to give to a friend. Words like, "Breathe" or "1–2–3" might be helpful, or a dark blue sky with tiny white dot stars and one arching yellow shooting star for the child to hold hopefulness with. A person close to the child who has died might have their name painted on the stone and then be held in the child's hand as a symbol of remembering the good times and memories.

Worry Dolls

Classic "Worry Dolls" are a Guatemalan staple that can be ordered online by a number of companies. Therapists and clients can create their own makeshift worry dolls by twisting part of a tissue into a tiny body shape and using tape to secure the sections. The little "dolls" can then be colored in, adding clothes and drawn-on faces. Little scraps of fabric can be used to glue on for "clothes" for the dolls if the child wants to get even more creative. "Dolls" can also just be simple stick figure drawings that are cut out and laminated. With the laminated doll version, a particular worry can be assigned to each doll by writing it on the laminate with a Dry Erase™ marker. This way, the problems assigned can change each week for the dolls to carry if need be.

Therapists can explain to child clients that the intention of worry dolls is to tell each one a particular fear or worry they have and then put it under their pillow at night and the doll will take care of the worry and when the clients wake up, they will feel less worried. Of course, there may be a placebo effect here, but in any case, the use of worry dolls is a playful way to address anxiety with young clients.

Message in a Bottle

Small glass bottles can be purchased in bulk online or therapists can collect tiny bottles from condiments or other items at home to be used for this activity. Home goods, department, or other decorating stores often have small bottles for sale as well. The idea behind this activity is that kid clients can write messages to themselves about hopes, goals, beliefs, and stuff them inside the bottles and tuck them away somewhere for future reading. I once had a 25-year-old man contact me as he was packing up his childhood room to move into his first apartment. He had found his "message in a bottle" from his time in therapy with me when he was 12 years old and reported having wept when he read his hopes for his grown up self. He shared that it was such a powerful experience for him and one he would do with his own children when he had them.

Story Bag

As described a bit in Chapter 6 as being useful in Narrative Therapy work, the "story bag" is one of the easiest games to incorporate into practice with younger clients. I use a silk drawstring bag for this activity, but any solid bag, box, or other container that a client cannot see into will work. Any random objects can be placed inside, so it's a good thing to clean out your junk drawers or children's playrooms for. The first five objects I pulled out just now from my story bag are a tiny, rubbery beige horse figurine, a pencil eraser shaped like a hamburger, an extra-large "cats eye" marble, a colorful butterfly iron-on patch, and a tiny doll hairbrush.

The story bag is used as a playful way to prompt (and control) conversations toward a therapeutic pathway. Chapter 6 gives a more detailed description, but in short, therapist and child take turns pulling one random object from the bag and creating a story together. If the child pulls the butterfly on their turn and weaves a tale of world takeover by the army of zombie butterflies (the "AZB"), the therapist can then take back control of the story by pulling the tiny hairbrush and stating,

> And then a magic hairbrush appeared and it's job was to comb out all the mean butterflies so only the beautiful, kind, sweet ones were left. And as the hairbrush did its job, it wondered what it would feel to be a butterfly and go to school each day with *only* nice, kind other butterflies?

Calming Clay

Any sort of pliable dough or clay can work for this activity, but my favorite brand is Model Magic™. Individual bags or tiny plastic cans of a single-colored substance can be purchased fairly inexpensively online. The other item needed for this is an assortment of scented essential oils. Good choices are lavender, lemon, rose, chamomile, or orange. This activity is best used with clients with anxiety or anger issues.

Therapists can let young clients choose a little bag or can of their preferred color of modeling clay. Next, they can choose which oil scent they like the best and the therapist can put a drop or two onto the clay and massage it in. Now, the child has a sensory object that they can get warm and malleable in their hand that has a calming smell to it. The therapist will then have the client use the clay as a calming tool during visualization or meditating exercises or during conversations that may bring up difficult emotions or anxiety for the child. The clay can be wrapped in plastic wrap or a small plastic bag and taken home for use whenever needed.

A note about essential oils: therapists should advise parents/caregivers about this activity in case the child has a rare allergy to the oil. Also, some oils, if not diluted properly, can be irritating to hands, so therapists should be mindful of checking concentrations of the oils and reading what amount to use and if it needs to be diluted before use to avoid being a possible irritant.

Therapeutic Games

Therapeutic games are plentiful to order online from a number of companies that supply therapists with therapeutic tools. There are many good ones, and new ones are being created every year. It's a wise idea to utilize what others have put time and effort and research into creating whenever possible. Although this book offers many playful interventions, therapeutic games can add yet another layer of helpful activities to the child-friendly therapy room.

Magnetic Words Expression

Therapists can order a number of different themed sets of magnetic words that are a fun way for kid clients to express their thoughts and feelings. These sets are available from a variety of companies online. It is also pretty easy for therapists to make their own, or have kid clients make their own sets of magnetic words. Doing the work of creating their own allows for personalization of words and themes that seem to fit best for therapists' specific client populations.

Craft, office supply, or chain retail stores will have rolls of magnetic strip. Using scissors, therapists can cut off tiny one-inch pieces and affix a small strip of self-adhesive paper or blank mailing or folder labels to the front of each. On the paper, therapists and clients can write words to use in meaningful ways. For example, include a range of subjects or people (I, you, he, they, dog, man, teacher, mother, stepfather, friend, bully, etc.), verbs (go, walk, fight, feel, talk, yell, hurt, cry), and adjectives (peacefully, quietly, loudly, angrily, calmly). Random "filler" words can be added as well and the collection can keep growing with each new client.

Therapists can ask kid clients to create sentences that describe how they are feeling or what has happened during the week. If family members are involved in sessions they can contribute as well or challenge certain words from the child's choice. For example, if 11-year-old Emily sticks the following words to the metal surface: *My mother fights with me angrily,* Emily's mom might add, "Was I really fighting 'angrily' Emily? Or was it more like 'frustratedly?'" The therapist can then help coach Emily and mom toward a better understanding of their arguments.

Dry-Erase Boards

A solid staple in any therapy room is a dry erase board and erasable markers. There are innumerable uses for these, including making lists, creating goals, drawing genograms (from Chapter 3), creating family contracts, or just random drawing. Some therapists write inspirational weekly messages on the board, while others might like (especially minimally talkative clients and families) to have clients or family members take turns going up and writing a goal for the session or the name of who they think should talk first, etc.

Bug Lollipops

Bug lollipops are available singly on line or cheaper as a bulk purchase. These are fully edible, clear, colored lollipops with a visible insect in the middle of it. You can buy them with things like crickets, ants, worms, and scorpions inside. The bug lollipops can be used as a really shocking, fun "gift" for a kid client who has made great progress, or used therapeutically as described below.

The lollipops can be an example of the concept of multiple views and context. Most children's first reaction to seeing the bug lollipops is something like, "Oh my gosh—ewwwww, that's so gross!" Therapists can help the child expand on their thoughts of why the lollipop is gross. Then the therapist can introduce the possibility of other people maybe *not* finding them gross. The therapist can then explain that in some cultures, certain bugs are a delicacy. And that to someone who is lost and stranded in the woods and starving, those bug lollipops would look pretty good. Adding this context can help kid clients better understand how different people might have different views of things *and* some of the reasons *why* they might feel differently than the client. This can be used as a jumping-off point for other topics of difference, like why one kid at school might not dress "cool" like the other kids or why one teacher is "mean" while the others or not.

A note on bug lollipops—these are not appropriate for all child clients. Therapists should thoroughly screen kid clients for vegetarianism, sensitivity to animals or insects, fears or allergies, and always check with parents/guardians first to be sure this seems like an appropriate activity.

15 Master List of Items for a Well-Stocked Child-Friendly Therapy Office

**Please note that this is a thorough range of items, varying in cost and space needs from small to large, but even the simplest, low cost or free items here can make for playful, effective therapy. Additionally many of these items are reusable with clients over and over again making them a one-time cost.

- A variety of coloring books, paper (construction, colored, white copier, and decorative print), crayons, markers, and other drawing supplies.
- Scrap paper or junk mail (to wad up and "make baskets" into the garbage can with when asking/answering questions as described in Chapter 14 activity.)
- Old magazines (to use in collage activities as described in Chapter 14).
- Bubble mailers (for remote kid clients as described in Chapter 14s section on sending teletherapy clients a "starter kit") These can be purchased in bulk on-line or in office supply or big, chain stores. They range from plain manila ones to a variety of brightly colored, themed, or holiday-styled ones. Stickers or colorful stamps can be used to decorate the outside of the mailers if plain ones are purchased.
- Extra-large popsicle sticks (to use for red light/green light activity in Chapter 14).
- Laminate sheets (to make worksheets or other print activities reusable) and Dry Erase™ or another brand of erasable markers to use on the laminated charts and sheets.
- Roll of peel-off magnetic tape (for Chapter 14 affirmations activity).
- Stickers.
- Assorted sequins, buttons, beads, or fake jewels (for decorating journals or soothing boxes).
- Tape, glue sticks, stapler.
- Rocks (preferably with a flat surface area), paints, paint pens, and acrylic sprays (to seal the paint and make it waterproof).
- Scissors (especially decorative edge ones).
- Sticky notes (in a variety of colors, sizes, and shapes).

DOI: 10.4324/9781003506072-16

- Journals (these can be ordered bulk online with a very wide range of pricing, or can be created by stapling together sheets of paper).
- Model Magic™ (or other soft, malleable dough or clay product).
- A variety of scented essential oils.
- Therapeutic games.
- A variety of "mindless" games (that don't require a lot of attention or thinking to facilitate therapeutic conversation while playing—Connect 4™).
- Simple puzzles (that families of children and therapists can work on together to practice things like patience, taking turns, communication, and teamwork).
- Tissues (for comfort and for balling up and throwing between therapist and client or family members in place of a talking stick).
- A soft ball that can tossed between people without risk of injury to people or objects in the therapy room.
- Bubbles (for the therapist to blow and for kid clients to catch and pop and answer questions).
- A dollhouse and dolls or other figurines that represent various ages, skin colors, body types, etc. As an easier, less expensive option, use plastic farm or jungle animal figures instead of human doll representations. Kids love choosing animals to represent people, so this is an added layer of fun to dollhouse enactments.
- Shoeboxes or other small boxes made of cardboard, wood, or plastic (to make "soothing boxes" out of in Chapter 14).
- Roll of colored masking tape (to use for "boundary work" in Chapter 1).
- A variety of figurines or animal representations (that can be used to demonstrate.
- A selection of big pillows (both for comfort and for children to cover their faces with if needed).
- Worry Dolls (many companies make different versions of the original Guatemalan "Worry Dolls," but therapists can easily make their own for a cheaper and more artistic option).
- Glass Bottles with cork stoppers (can be ordered bulk online).
- Random small items (like the sorts of things one would get from those plastic capsules with prizes inside that come from gumball-type machines) for the story bag activity in Chapter 14.
- Bug lollipops (for Chapter 10, activity on perception and Chapter 14 activity on multiple points of view).
- Small, plastic blocks or "bricks" (like Legos™) to be used in various activities (e.g., Chapter 11 "Toxic Positivity" breakdown lane activity).
- Toy cars (for mindless play, or to represent people like in Chapter 11).

I'm sure that other experienced child and family therapists have created a million additional therapeutic activities and games for their younger clients, so the aforementioned list is limited to my personal tried-and-true favorites. I strongly encourage therapists to ask other therapists they know or work with about effective strategies for playful work with younger clients. Playful concepts are endless and it is always a good idea to keep a fresh stream of ideas on activities coming in.

References

Beck, A.T., Rush, A.J., Shaw, B.F., & Emery, G. (1979). *Cognitive therapy of depression.* Guilford Press.

Boszormenyi-Nagy, I. (1987). *Foundations of contextual therapy: Collected papers of Ivan Boszormenyi-Nagy.* Routledge. https://doi.org/10.4324/9781315803852

Bowen, M. (1966). The use of family theory in clinical practice. *Comprehensive Psychiatry, 7*(5), 345–374. https://doi.org/10.1016/S0010-440X(66)80065-2

Bratton, S.C., Ray, D., Rhine, T., & Jones, L. (2005). The efficacy of play therapy with children: A meta-analytic review of treatment outcomes. *Professional Psychology: Research and Practice, 36*(4), 376–390. https://doi.org/10.1037/0735-7028.36.4.376

Buckingham M., & Clifton, D.O. (2001). *Now, discover your strengths.* The Free Press.

Center for Substance Abuse Treatment (1999). *Brief interventions and brief therapies for substance abuse.* Rockville, MD: Substance Abuse and Mental Health Services Administration, US. (Treatment Improvement Protocol (TIP) Series, No. 34.) Available from: https://www.ncbi.nlm.nih.gov/books/NBK64947/

Dana, D. (2018). *The polyvagal theory in therapy: Engaging the rhythm of regulation.* W.W. Norton & Co.

de Shazer, S. (1982). *Patterns of family therapy: An ecosystemic approach.* Guilford Press.

Friedberg, R.D. (2006). A cognitive behavioral approach to family therapy. *Journal of Contemporary Psychotherapy, 36*(4), 159–165. https://doi.org/10.1007/s10879-006-9020-2

Haley, J. (1976). *Problem-solving therapy: New strategies for effective family therapy.* Jossey-Bass.

Jensen, S.A., Graham, E.R., & Biesen, J.N. (2017). A meta-analytic review of play therapy with emphasis on outcome measures. *Professional Psychology: Research and Practice, 48*(5), 390–400. https://doi.org/10.1037/pro0000148

Madanes, C. (1981). *Strategic family therapy.* Jossey-Bass.

Minuchin, S. (1974). *Families and family therapy.* Harvard University Press.

Niemec, R.M. (2018). *Character strengths interventions: A field guide for practitioners.* Hogrefe.

Perls, F., Hefferline, R.F., & Goodman, P. (1951). *Gestalt therapy: Excitement and growth in the human personality.* Julian Press.

Pinsof, W.M., Breunlin, D.C., Russell, W.P., Lebow, J., & Chambers, A.L. (2018). *Integrative systemic therapy: Metaframeworks for problem-solving with individuals, couples, and families.* American Psychological Association. https://doi.org/10.1037/0000055-000

Russell, W.P., Breunlin, D.C., & Sahebi, B. (2023). *Integrative systemic therapy in practice: A clinician's handbook.* Routledge, Taylor and Francis.

Sohol, M., Singh, P., Dhillon, B.S., & Gill, H.S. (2022). Efficacy of journaling in the management of mental illness: a systematic review and meta-analysis. *Family Medicine and Community Health, 10*(1), 1–7. https://doi.org/10.1136/fmch-2021-001154

Tuttle, L.C. (2003). Experiential family therapy: An innovative approach to the resolution of family conflict in genetic counseling. *Journal of Genetic Counseling, 7*(2), 167–186. https://doi.org/10.1023/A:1022802006630

White, M., & Epston, D. (1990). *Narrative means to therapeutic ends.* W. W. Norton & Company.

Index

For Product Safety Concerns and Information please contact our EU
representative GPSR@taylorandfrancis.com
Taylor & Francis Verlag GmbH, Kaufingerstraße 24, 80331 München, Germany

www.ingramcontent.com/pod-product-compliance
Lightning Source LLC
Chambersburg PA
CBHW070343270326
41926CB00017B/3962